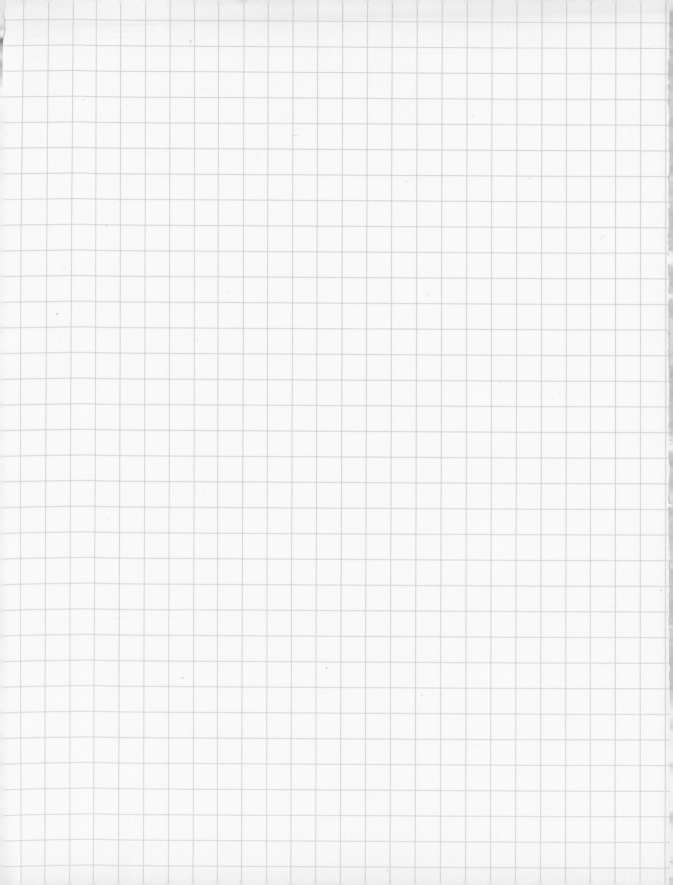

MUMMIN' IT

For Reuben, Tobias and Edith.

When I no longer hold your hands,
know you'll always hold my heart.

An Hachette UK Company
www.hachette.co.uk

First published in the Great Britain in
2021 by Kyle Books, an imprint of
Octopus Publishing Group Limited
Carmelite House
50 Victoria Embankment
London EC4Y 0DZ
www.kylebooks.co.uk

Text copyright
© Harriet Shearsmith 2021
Design and layout copyright
© Octopus Publishing Group Limited 2021

Publisher **Joanna Copestick**
Design **Helen Bratby**
Illustrations **Amy Blackwell**
Editor **Jenny Dye**
Production **Allison Gonsalves**

ISBN 978-0-85783-937-4

A CIP catalogue record for this book
is available from the British Library.

Printed and bound in China

10 9 8 7 6 5 4 3 2 1

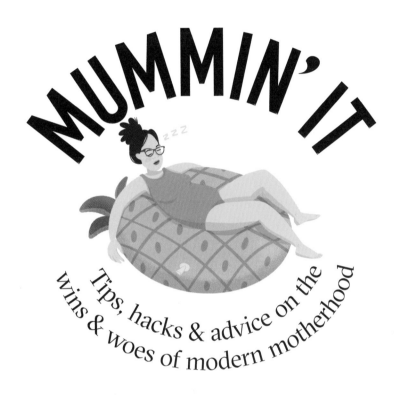

MUMMIN' IT

Tips, hacks & advice on the wins & woes of modern motherhood

Harriet Shearsmith

Kyle Books

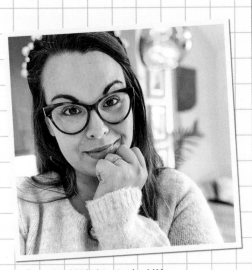

Based in Yorkshire in the UK, **HARRIET SHEARSMITH** runs her award-winning Toby & Roo blog from home. She is a breath of fresh air in the parenting world, where mothers can relate to her hacks which are aimed at simplifying everyday life while raising a smile. With over 100k dedicated Instagram followers, she reaches 1–2 million people each month across all her platforms and offers indispensable tips for busy working mums to help get them through each day.

www.tobyandroo.com
Instagram: @tobyandroo

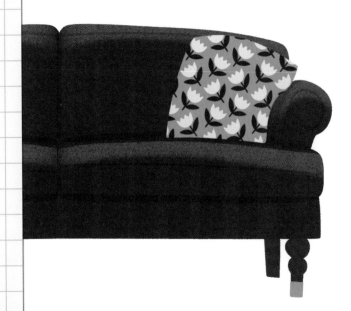

contents

welome to my world...

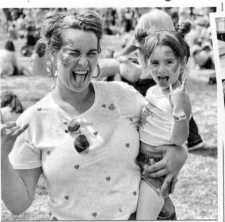
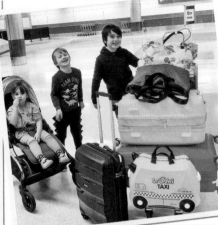
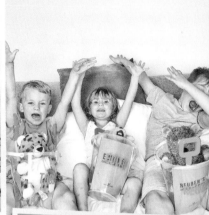
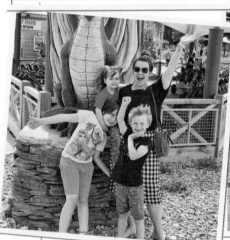
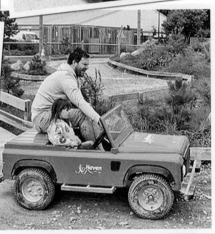
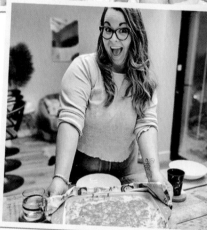
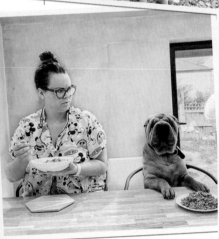
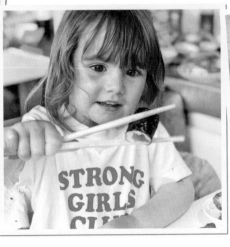
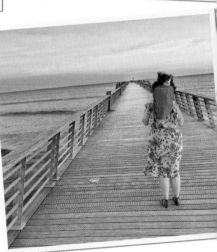

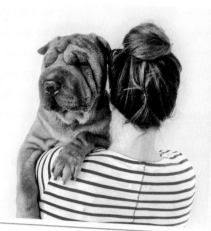
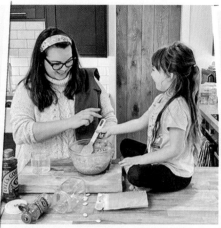
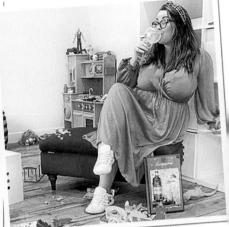
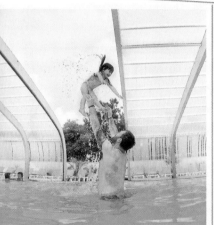
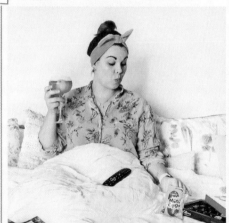
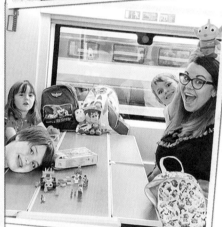
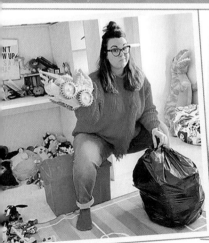
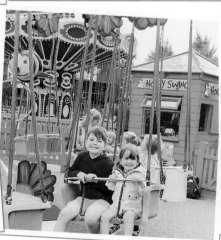
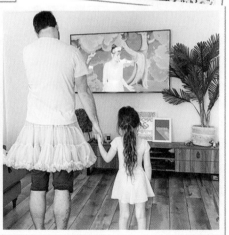

'Give me that backkkkkkk!' I can hear them bickering over their toys in the background while I try to get a little bit of work done, but to be honest I don't have the energy to shout **'Stoppppp bloodyyyyy fightinggggg!'** one more time today. And it's only 12.52 pm. I'm tired, I have deadlines and the house looks as if a bull that has been stung by a wasp has rampaged through it. A bull with a particular fancy for L.O.L dolls and Barbies.

Before I had kids, I remember everyone telling me that motherhood was the most rewarding thing they had ever done, that it was hard but 'oh so worth it'. What they didn't tell me was quite HOW hard it can be. How some days it can feel utterly incapacitating to be a mother, a wife, a worker and everything in between. When your new bundle arrives, you're given somewhat of a free pass, aren't you? 'Ooh don't be too hard on yourself, the laundry can wait,' they say. But it won't wait forever, will it? How long can you really go with no clean pants... a question I wouldn't dream of pushing any new mum to try and answer.

The thing is, what they don't tell you is that modern motherhood is the lifestyle equivalent of someone cooking a recipe and going freestyle. They have all the ingredients life is supposed to have, but then they get handy. Sprinkle in a bit of workplace pressure and inflexibility, add a teaspoon of wanting that modern, Pinterest-style house, a dash of 'does my partner still fancy me?' and a shaving of mum guilt on top.

In short, modern motherhood can be a bit of a bitch.

Of course, it can also be wonderful, and I do love it. But that is not why I have written this book. **It's not full of the lovely, fluffy mumsy stuff that you can find on any #blessed instagram post.** What I want to share with you is all the solid, practical tips that have seen me through the first ten years of life as a mother of three children and helped me survive. All these things have enabled me to see the wonderful when my eyes have been twitching from the difficult.

Mummin' It is filled with tips, hacks, advice and personal experiences that I hope will help make your life just that little bit simpler so you can focus on all the things that make motherhood and being a modern woman genuinely rewarding. Keep it on your coffee table or book shelf, and please don't feel the pressure to find 30 minutes to read it with a coffee as this is probably an unrealistic fantasy. I've deliberately designed it so you can dip in and out. Flick to the checklists in the travel section before you go abroad, earmark that hack for getting your oven spotless after the birthday cake (you felt pressured to bake) exploded in there or you left the casserole in too long (because you needed to answer a work email)... however you use it, this book is for you.

From one mother to another.

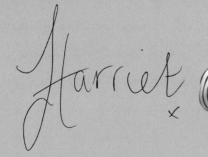

Harriet
x

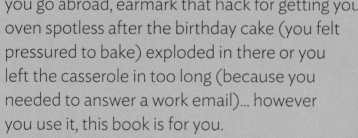

FOOD

I love food. I love to eat it, talk it, cook it, dream about it – my bedtime therapy is to watch endless food videos on Instagram before I doze off. I save them with absolutely every intention of trying them out one day, but I rarely do. In fact, I really ought to give that a go...

Food is a huge part of my life. As a serial snacker on the sofa, as a wife who loves a good dinner date, and as a mum who's greeted every afternoon post school with: **'Hi mum, what's for dinner?'**. I could go on and on, culminating in the ultimate food glory that is a takeaway in bed, but I will spare you the trauma of giving you that mental image in too much detail.

Fortunately for me, I've always loved cooking. I think it comes from my own mum and grandma's love of cooking. I admit I have none of their artistic flare for crafting a rose out of icing or making a birthday cake that doesn't suggest that its baker maybe had one too many gins before the decoration phase. **No, I'm not a pretty cook, but I am a good and enthusiastic cook** and am never afraid to take the whole family with me on a foray into the culinary unknown. This means that I have two children who are largely willing to try anything, and I have Edith, who is my curveball child. Her diet largely consists of pasta, chips, chocolate and my sanity. Getting her to try new things is becoming a little easier as she gets older, but it requires constant cajoling, much muttered swearing and the occasional shouted **'will you just eat it!!!'** – all the things those parenting experts tell you not to do.

Even as a baby, Edith was always the one who would rather have 'boobie' than anything else and, like most kids who are third or fourth or fifth in line, her first taste of food was a far cry from the homemade purées I made for her siblings. In fact, it was a chip, slipped to her by my eldest, Reuben, when mummy was trying to get Toby to sit still. From then on, it became a thing – if she saw chips on other people's plates, she would bounce and reach. We have since pipped chips to the post as a favourite food, replacing them with the equally beige pasta. I can confirm that she still refers to green food and herbs as 'leaves'. One of the things I have learnt with Edith and her fussiness is to roll with it. When she was smaller it would always cause me such stress – why didn't she love food the way the rest of us did? Am I sure she is mine? Now, we have a rule of trying something and if it's really not liked, that's OK. Does it always work? Of course not, but we try and I don't stress out when she isn't playing ball.

Despite the challenges meal times can sometimes hold for us as parents, they still remain one of my favourite times of the day. We all come together and talk about what we did during our days, what we enjoyed, what we didn't. It's a time to regroup as a family, a time to hit the pause button on everything, if only for 20 minutes or so. Even when meal times don't involve the family or a home cooked meal, food will always be a love in my life.

Now I have filled you with excitement at the prospect of taking cookery and family food tips from me, **I think we should probably just get on with it, don't you?**

Meal planning

If you had told me at the age of nineteen that I was one day going to be excited about sitting down and creating a weekly meal plan, I would have laughed at you. Literally howled as I swaggered away in my teeny tiny skirt. Yet here we are. Not only am I thrilled by meal plans, but I've included a nice chunky section on meal planning in this book. And this is why – it will change your family life for the better. It will save you time, money and sanity. Three pretty big things, in my eyes.

Why would I meal plan, Harriet?

There are so many reasons. Initially, I was sceptical. What if we didn't fancy Spag Bol on Tuesday, or we went out for an impromptu dinner one night? However, I've realised that planning ahead gives you a structure and there is also flexibility in it. Of course, things don't always go to plan and you can use up any leftover food the following week to cut down on waste.

TIME

There is something liberating about knowing what you're having for dinner. Whether you work at home or another location, you're always going to be busy and suddenly that dinner hour creeps up on you and BAM, you're faced with a horde of hungry people. You're hungry too but strangely, as you stare into the fridge, nothing inspires you. Everything feels like it takes too long or is too complicated and all you can do is reach for the pasta again. However, if you put a stew on the meal plan, you know that you need to whack it in the slow cooker, so perhaps you do it in the morning and then there it is, right when you need it, at the end of a long day. Maybe you know that on a Wednesday you have gymnastics club after school, or you have a meeting at work until late, so having something pre-prepared is invaluable. Alternatively, you can do something simple, like beans on toast or a stir-fry that takes minutes to throw together. Whatever the meal, planning it will save you time.

MONEY

It will also save you money – moola, skrilla, dosh. Whatever you call it, we all want to save it for more important meals, like a Friday night takeaway, or that meal you've been looking forward to with the girls. Planning meals can save you a lot of money in two ways:

Firstly, you only buy what you need and don't overdo it. If you're not nipping to the shop for that 'one thing' (that turns into multiple things) that you need for a recipe, you'll spend far less in the long run.

Secondly, you save money because you can adhere to a strict budget. If you only have a certain amount to spend on food shopping each week then you can tailor a meal plan to that effect. There are some wonderful blogs and books out there that can give you recipes for as little as a pound or two per family of four. If you're strapped, meal planning really is your essential tool.

ENCOURAGES EXPLORATION

Meal planning also hauls you out of those meal ruts. My other half, Adam, once turned to me just after dinner and, in the sort of voice you would use to approach a wild animal, he said, 'Do you mind if we have something different for tea tomorrow?' After a bit of yelling about how Adam should cook his own bloody dinner if he didn't like my meals, I worked out that we had been eating the same six meals on rotation for weeks and weeks. I had got stuck on all the things I knew the kids would eat and the things I knew how to cook well. While I wouldn't say that is a major issue, it's really good to switch it up every so often. There will be evenings when you try a meal and you think 'all that effort and no one liked it' – but you tried it, you explored something new and you can make a note that it's not the one. And similarly, there will be nights when you strike gold, when they exclaim, 'We love it!' and the feeling of satisfaction that brings is just the best.

ENVIRONMENT

Yes, meal planning is good for the environment. No, I haven't just pulled that out of my arse, it's true! It leads to less waste and waste is bad for the environment.

NUMBER 1 TIP FOR MEAL PLANNING: Accept that some nights it won't go to plan and that's ok! Use last week's 'fails' as this week's 'wins' – create a meal this week out of leftovers from last week.

TOP TIP

If you're really keen to focus on the environment with your meal plans, you can find out if there are any refill/zero waste shops near you where you can (sometimes) take your own container and ditch the packaging altogether. You can get rice, pasta, pulses and spices and they're often a lot cheaper too. Try searching your location on **zerowastenear.me**

So, what is the best way to meal plan for a family?

I feel like a bit of a wally telling someone 'how' to meal plan – it's not rocket science and maybe you're thinking that I'm a bit of a patronising cow. However, over the years, I've discovered a few best practices when it comes to meal planning that have helped me stay on track.

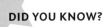

DID YOU KNOW?

If you are an online food shopper, then check out whether your supermarket of choice offers a scheme where you pay a monthly subscription and your deliveries are free. It can save you quite a bit each month.

LOOK AT WHO AND WHEN

Sounds daft, but it's not. In our house, we have five people who would normally sit down for dinner between 5 and 6 pm. Now, if that actually happened every night then it would all be a doddle, but that isn't the reality of family life. On at least one evening, Toby has football practice and then eats with Adam on the way home and so, on those days, I don't have to think about what those two might like/not like.

Always look at who is going to be home and when, then plan accordingly. Need something fast because you don't get home until 5.30 pm and they are all famished? Great, then you need a meal that is either done and waiting for you or can be ready in under 15 minutes. Everyone's at home and you have a bit of time to spare? Then you can choose something with longer prep.

DON'T LET AGE HOLD YOU BACK

To elaborate – don't let your kids' ages hold you back. I learnt with Toby, that once he started weaning, I didn't need to do something different for him. If we were eating a casserole, I would simply purée some for him. If we were eating a Sunday roast, he would have some veggies and Yorkshire pudding as finger food. It was so liberating to realise that I didn't need to cook different things for him or waste money on pouches for the house. (I bought them for when we were out and about because they were SO much easier.)

TRY SOMETHING NEW EACH WEEK

If you want to force yourself out of your comfort zone and even enjoy a little creativity, then try something new every week. It could be that you want to try and cut back on your meat consumption, so a Meatless Monday is your chance to try a vegetarian recipe, or it might be that you want to try a specific food you haven't before, like jackfruit. It could even be that you want to cook something fairly standard but try a recipe you have never done before. Whatever tickles your pickle, use your meal planning to make it happen once a week.

UTILISE PINTEREST

Ahh Pinterest, the place where our dreams of gloriously designed pantries and beautiful craft projects are held. While Pinterest seems like a place that is utterly unrealistic, it's actually my favourite place to find recipes. The internet has replaced cook books and magazines as my number one spot to grab new ideas for dinners and Pinterest is my Google of food. I type in things like 'vegetarian meals in 15 minutes' or 'chicken casserole recipes' or 'quick family meals' and it always delivers. And the best part is that it's always being updated!

DO THE SHOPPING AS YOU GO

If you're someone who gets their food delivered, I recommend you do your online shop at the same time as you plan your meals. You can select a recipe, check the cupboard and then add the necessary ingredients to your order. If you don't shop online, you can still write your shopping list as you plan.

ALWAYS CHECK YOUR CUPBOARDS AND SEARCH RECIPES BY INGREDIENTS

Remember what I said about cutting down on waste? The easiest way to do this is to check your cupboards and work from there. Typing into Pinterest 'recipes using XYZ' will often yield results that will help you use up the products from the deep dark depths of your cupboard. It helps you save space in your kitchen too!

DON'T FORGET TO WRITE DOWN WHERE YOU FOUND THE RECIPE

Nothing is more annoying than buying all the ingredients and then having no idea where you got the recipe. It's just not what you need at 4 pm on a Monday afternoon when you're trying to crack on with dinner. Make a note on your meal plan of where to find your recipe (even if that is a link saved in your phone's notes).

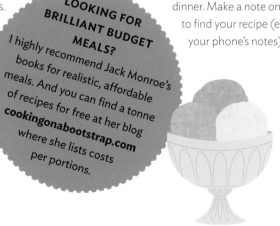

LOOKING FOR BRILLIANT BUDGET MEALS? I highly recommend Jack Monroe's books for realistic, affordable meals. And you can find a tonne of recipes for free at her blog **cookingonabootstrap.com** where she lists costs per portions.

Meal plan

MONDAY

SPAGHETTI BOLOGNESE WITH HIDDEN VEG

I make as usual and then grate in a carrot and courgette and finely chop mushrooms and peppers! They'll never know!

TUESDAY

FISH FINGERS & STUFFED PEPPERS

tobyandroo.com

WEDNESDAY

15 MIN CHICKEN STIR FRY

ohsweetbasil.com

THURSDAY

CHICKEN SATAY SKEWERS WITH PEANUT DIP SERVED WITH RICE

Marinade in the morning or night before
tobyandroo.com

FRIDAY

TAKEAWAY

SATURDAY

GREEN THAI CURRY

I use green Thai curry paste for ease and finely slice veg like carrots, courgettes, mange tout and peppers into the sauce

SUNDAY

VEGETABLE LASAGNE

thecookreport.com

Meal plan

DATE 08/11

MONDAY

BEEF & LENTIL COTTAGE PIE WITH CAULIFLOWER & POTATO TOPPING

Great for freezer portions **bbcgoodfood.com**

TUESDAY

MACARONI CHEESE

WEDNESDAY

PRESSURE COOKER CHICKEN ENCHILADAS

number2pencil.com

THURSDAY

GINGER CHICKEN MEATBALLS IN PEANUT SAUCE

Make the night before because of after school club

ambitiouskitchen.com

FRIDAY

TAKEAWAY

Adam collect on way home from football

SATURDAY

HOMEMADE PIZZA

Make dough in the morning

SUNDAY

CHICKEN, BACON & MUSHROOM PIE WITH MASH AND VEG

kitchensanctuary.com

THESE ARE SAMPLE MEAL PLANS
Head to page 202 and jot down your own meal plans.

Budgeting the meal plan

Saving money and sticking to a budget is such a huge advantage of meal planning that it's important, I feel, to go all the way. So, here are a few more tips.

DITCH THE BRANDS

Ditch brands and shop the supermarket-own range. I tried this last week as a comparative shop and you know how much I saved? Enough for a ticket at the cinema. Not even joking. The pennies on each item quickly accumulate into pounds, and there is often not much difference in the taste or quality of the product, or at least not enough difference to be an issue for you if you are trying to cut costs. If that doesn't sound like much, then multiply it by 52 weeks in the year!

STICK TO THE SIMPLE

A bugbear of mine is that often the recipes that I want to try, which are something a bit 'different', are the ones that are the most expensive. We found an absolutely wonderful gumbo recipe that was truly unusual and everyone loved it. However, unfortunately, it was damned expensive to make. Sticking to simpler but nutritionally balanced meals is often a good idea if you are trying to cut cost.

MAKE IT, DON'T BUY IT

Time is a luxury and something most of us don't have, so while this is something to bear in mind, it might not be an easy option for the majority of us who are busy working our arses off. IF you can, making things, like bread, is a lot cheaper than buying it, as is making stock and using every last bit of your food. Again, we're talking time-intensive so it might not be for you, but on those chilled Sunday mornings maybe have a go at making some bread with the kids. It's a double whammy as not only does it save you some pennies, it also keeps them entertained (for approximately 4 minutes until they get bored and leave you to finish it off alone).

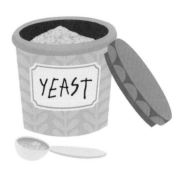

TOP TIP Ask the bakery section in your local supermarket if they have any fresh yeast you can have – they often give it to you for freeeee!

PRE-EMPTIVE SHOPPING

There are two ways to do this – if you're an online shopper, then look at what items are on offer before you create your meal plan. If you're an in-store shopper, head straight to the reduced section, buy a selection of items and then build meals around that. It doesn't always work, as frequently the only things you will find in the reduced section are ready meals and things you can't really use, but it can occasionally be useful.

CHANGE UP YOUR MEATS
OR DITCH THEM ALTOGETHER

Second only to household cleaning products (the killer on my weekly shop), I would recommend changing your meats or ditching them completely. Thighs instead of breasts, turkey instead of beef mince, changing out beef for veggies in recipes. Quorn is actually more expensive, but beans are cheap in comparison to beef and make a lush lentil and bean stew.

after the meal plan...

So now you have your meal plan and that's it, right?

Well, yes and no. Yes, most likely you're a full grown adult who can work out how to cook stuff for themselves and doesn't need me to tell you what to do with a meal plan that you have created. And no, because every day I read a new mum hack somewhere or someone shares something online about what they do to make their lives easier and simpler and I just didn't think of it. Every day really is a school day.

So, while that might be the end of my 'meal plan tips', I thought it was the perfect prelude to some ideas for how to make your kitchen a simpler and thus happier place.

The kitchen hotlist

You know how you have those celeb hotlists? Well, this is the same but, you know, for kitchens. Less 'thirsty' and more *actually thirsty*. Beyond the everyday products that we all have in our kitchen, these are the extras that I value for making my life so much easier.

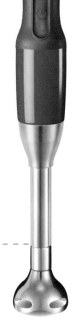

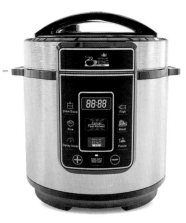

PRESSURE COOKER

I can't begin to express to you how much I love my pressure cooker – it is a love affair Disney wishes it had written – and it's first on the list because it is the one that I use most often. I'd recommend a pressure cooker over a slow cooker any day and if you invest in a decent one that has a slow cooker setting, you have two functions in one. I have the Pressure King Pro (sounds kinky) and it's excellent. It's also worth pointing out that when we had our extension and no kitchen for weeks and weeks on end, this was a life saver; a small kitchen all in one. It fries, it bakes, it slow-cooks and it does it all at super-speed.

HAND BLENDER

One of the things that I have learnt to do over the years is blend veggies into Edith's food. The poor kid is oblivious that she is being fed the good stuff against her will. Insert evil laugh here. In the past, I always had a food blender but, when we did up the kitchen, I got rid of it and found that my hand blender is better, cheaper and easier to use. If you're making smoothies and such, you probably still want a proper blender, or at the very least a hand blender with attachments, but for soups and sauces a little hand blender, such as this one from Kitchen Aid, is the tool to have.

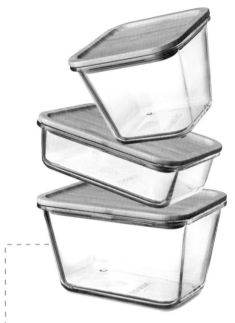

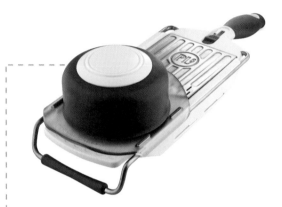

MANDOLINE SLICER

This is a nifty little tool that cuts, slices, dices, cubes, mashes and shreds your food, thus making meal prep ridiculously easy. Everything is done in minutes and, when you're hard-pressed for time, this is an amazing thing. Best of all? You can bag a decent one, such as this mandoline slicer from Oxo, for a reasonable price. No more smearing the mascara as you try to chop onions.

MICROWAVE RICE COOKER

Yes, you can cook rice in a saucepan, but my family has enjoyed much more since we got a microwave rice cooker. I bang in a cup of rice, stick it in the microwave and out it comes – flawless, fluffy rice. It frees up my hob for cooking other things and means I'm not having to monitor anything. They start from as little as £10.

FOOD STORAGE

When I first saw the internet's obsession with food storage, it just seemed a bit daft to me. However, it's actually made a huge difference to our kitchen and how easily I find things. Before I decanted my shopping into its 'correct' containers and just kept the pasta or rice in the bag that it arrived in, I would pull everything out, spill things and generally make a huge mess and get really annoyed. Having food storage makes life so much easier as everything is a similar size and fits into your cupboards much more neatly. Ikea are food storage champions, but there are so many places you can go to. Pro tip: You can use these in your fridge too for things like cheese – grate your cheese to make things speedier.

The 'How do we get them to eat it?!' section

Excellent, you've planned the meal and filled the kitchen with all the wonderful things that make cooking for your little darlings a doddle. They arrive home from school, ravenous beasts loudly declaring that they are starrrrrvvving, despite having eaten a snack in the car. You have lovingly prepared their food and present it to them to be met with… **'I don't like it'.**
Well. That pissed on your bonfire didn't it?

Undoubtedly, every parent will have been faced with this phrase. For me, it's infrequent with the boys but a favourite phrase of Edith's. The most infuriating part is that, even before there's time to sniff the meal, she declares her dissatisfaction. It's an almost instantaneous case of 'I don't know it, therefore I don't like it'. On the odd occasion, she will throw me a bone and declare something as 'dewishwus' (that's delicious to you and me), taking me completely by surprise. However, a good 90 per cent of the time, it's a battle that ranges from 'I don't like that' to 'I'm full' after merely half a spoonful or one unenthusiastic lick.

So how do you get kids to eat the things you put in front of them?

This is something that the experts simply can't seem to agree on. Some will tell you it's just a phase and to wait it out, keep persevering but make sure that you have another option set aside so that your child isn't hungry. Others will tell you that you need to be firm, offer no alternatives and simply carry on.

Most of us, if we're honest, sit somewhere in the middle. No one wants the trauma of a hungry child whinging like a wildebeest that stood on a thorn after a long hard day, but very few of us want to be functioning as a restaurant every evening, cooking up an array of dishes while our own miniature Gordon Ramsay barks at us to hurry up. Some days, I just don't have it in me to argue and I will end up doing a slice of bread for Edith after she's tried the obligatory few mouthfuls of food (nutritional, I know). Most nights, however, I am the mean mummy who insists she finishes the majority of her bowl or she will eat nothing at all. It's finding a balance between good cop and bad cop and finding what works for you as a family and as a parent.

Here are a few things that work for me:

BALANCE IT OUT
Try to cook meals that you know they love and will eat (so, beige ones) and then mix it up another night with something that they haven't tried before.

HIDE THE GOOD STUFF
Veggies and fruit are considered one of the more sinister things that the Earth has to offer in Edith's book. Hiding them in sauces is a winner, everything from grated carrots and courgettes in tomato sauces to finely chopped celery, grated carrot and minced broccoli in a cottage pie. If she can't see it, she usually doesn't even notice. A few months ago, I hit my sneaky peak when I managed to chop pineapple and peppers so finely and melt them down in the sauce so that she could only pucker her brow as the flavours hit. She ate everything and, as you can imagine, I revelled in a smugness that only comes from getting one over on your kid.

LET THEM HELP YOU COOK
I know a lot of you will probably feel like this is the least helpful suggestion in the world because NOTHING makes you want to scream, 'Will you just let me do it!!' than a child massacring a carrot or a pepper. But, and it's a pretty big but, despite the extra time it will of course add to the cooking, there are a bajillion (maybe a vague exaggeration) studies that suggest that children are more likely to eat the things that they cook. I guess it removes the mystery of the food. We don't do it all the time but, during the school holidays or at weekends, it can be really useful and effective.

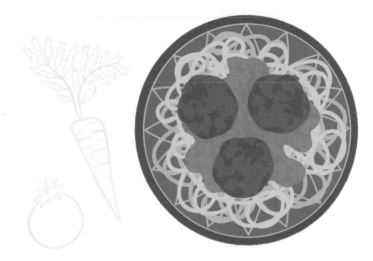

PICKY LUNCHES

These are a popular tool in our house for getting them to at least try something. It's a bit like the party buffet where you take a tablespoon of dubious-looking rice or couscous, knowing full well that you should have just stuck to the cold pizza and vol-au-vents. I pack several small tapas dishes with all sorts of things and then pop it on the table and leave it. I rarely find anything left, and I will often see Edith or Toby picking up something they haven't tried before because they have a fear of missing out on the latest treat. It doesn't always work, but I've also been known to say, 'If you're hungry and there is food still in the dishes, you can go finish that first'.

BE FIRM

We have a rule: try a few mouthfuls and, if you really don't like it, then fine. You don't have to finish your bowl, but you won't get a replacement meal. Ninety-nine per cent of the time, Edith does come around and eats some of her dinner, at least enough to placate me and remove the risk of hunger. As adults, I think we also forget that sometimes you just aren't that keen or you aren't in the mood for what you've been offered and that is OK. It's getting them to try it that is the most important thing.

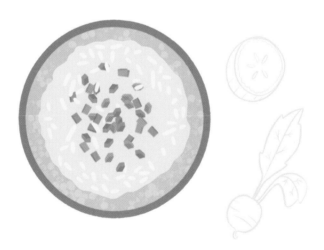

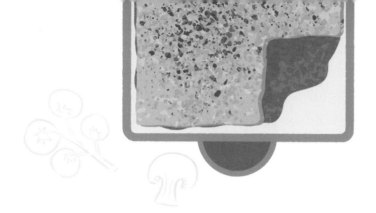

NO TREATS

This is what I meant when I said I will sometimes cave and give Edith a slice of bread after a long day. A slice of bread is not a treat, whereas if I want her to eat her dinner but she can smell my weakness and knows that her alternative option is a packet of sweets or her beloved Barney bears, then she isn't going to entertain me. By making her 'substitute' something she really isn't that fussed about, she will weigh up the pros and cons in her noggin before commencing jaw lockdown.

PUT THE UNKNOWN IN THE KNOWN

You know when you just *know* a meal and you're comfortable with it? Children are exactly the same; there will be some meals that they just know and feel safe with. Pasta is one for Edith – as fussy as she can be, she loves pasta and always has. Slowly introducing the unknown into her pasta meals has been really useful. She will eat things that I know she wouldn't touch if I was giving them to her in another manner. You can try it with anything that you know they like!

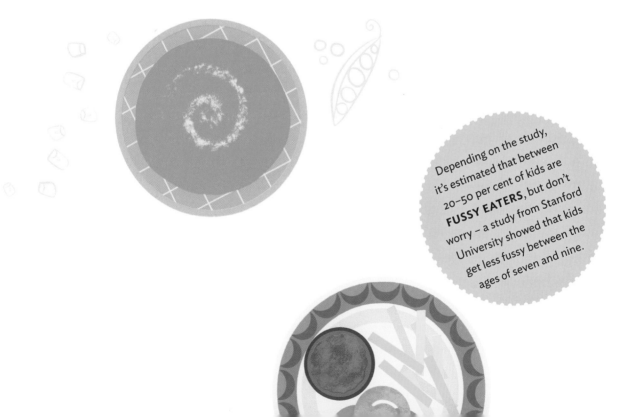

Depending on the study, it's estimated that between 20–50 per cent of kids are **FUSSY EATERS**, but don't worry – a study from Stanford University showed that kids get less fussy between the ages of seven and nine.

Homemade chicken nuggets with hidden treasure

AND BY TREASURE, I MEAN VEG! ———→

Simple, easy and familiar to most children, but with lots of hidden goodness!

Makes 12 nuggets

INGREDIENTS

1 courgette, peeled and grated

1 carrot, finely grated

2 chicken breasts or thighs

90g sweetcorn

2 tablespoons onion granules or
  1 small onion, peeled and
  finely chopped

2–3 tablespoons plain flour

1 egg, beaten

150g panko breadcrumbs

dash of oil (around 1 tablespoon)

salt and freshly ground black pepper

1. Squeeze the excess moisture out of the courgette and carrot.

2. In a food processor, blend together the chicken, vegetables and onion granules until smooth. Season with salt and pepper.

3. Form the mixture into small nugget or croquette shapes (it should make roughly 12), then dip each nugget into the flour, followed by the egg and finally the panko breadcrumbs, to coat.

4. Add a dash of oil to your pan, place over a high heat and then fry the nuggets for 3 minutes on each side, until golden and cooked through. I like to serve with bread and butter (my kids will almost always make themselves a sandwich... they do it with everything!). Sometimes we will have chips or wedges as well.

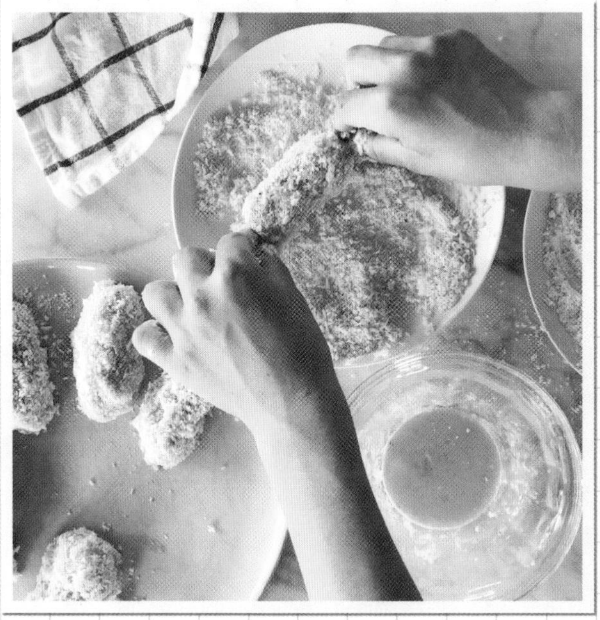

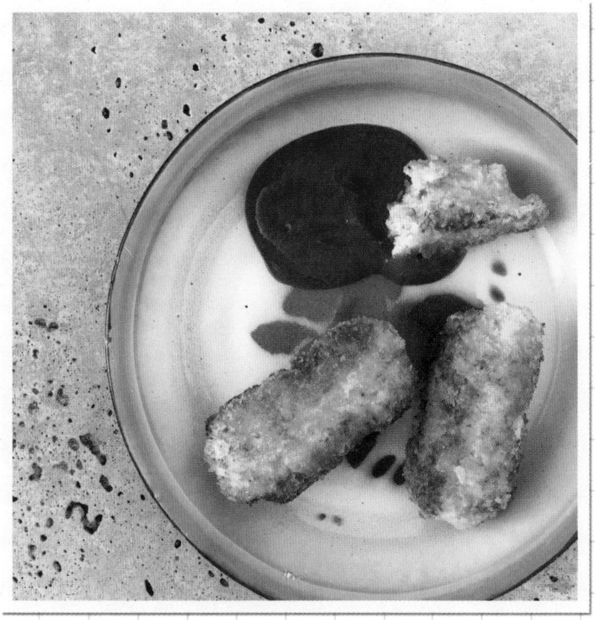

Mum's meal bingo

See how many you can tick off through the course of a meal – we've all been there. The temper tantrums over the wrong bowl, the cold leftovers you know you shouldn't eat but you polish off anyway... go on, have a giggle and know you aren't alone.

Child had a temper tantrum or cried because you gave them the wrong plate.

Child asked about dinner before you got a hello after school or preschool.

You said, 'You won't get any pudding!', knowing full well you hadn't made any anyway.

You broke up an argument over who sits where at the dinner table.

You ate your child's cold leftovers.

Child refused to eat something that they absolutely devoured last week on the grounds that they 'don't like it'.

You drank the rest of the wine you were cooking with.

You muttered, 'I don't know why I bother' under your breath.

You fed the kids one meal and then ate by yourself or with a partner after their bed, just so you can eat in peace.

You made enough pasta to serve an army... or far too little.

You said, 'I told you that you wouldn't eat your dinner if you kept having snacks.'

You lied about what is in the meal just to avoid an argument... 'Mushrooms? No darling, I wouldn't dream of it.'

You all ate dinner in front of the TV, just for ease.

You had a dinnertime plan and ditched it all for a takeaway because you had a bad day.

You discovered your child eats something at school that they flatly refuse to try at home.

You cleaned up a drink spill that you *just* warned them was going to happen.

DID YOU GET BINGO? If it's been an especially bad day, you can always turn this into a drinking game; down a shot for every one you manage to get – though, to be honest, it's probably not worth the hangover with the kids.

Making food more fun

Over the last few years there has been a huge rise in the use of things like bento boxes and funky little cutters for kids' sandwiches. I was at first resistant to filling the kitchen with lots of useless bits and pieces but, in fact, I've found many of them to be rather clever.

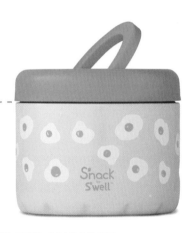

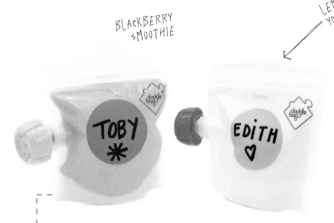

BLACKBERRY SMOOTHIE

LEMON YOGURT

INSULATED CONTAINER

You know how you might take leftovers to work the following day for lunch? Well, why is it that we never do that for our kids? If I had a penny for every time I heard a parent say, 'But he doesn't really like sandwiches' or 'Urgh, the whole sandwich came back with just one mouthful bitten out, no wonder she's starving!'... well let's just say I would be writing this book from an island in the Maldives. There are loads of child-friendly insulated container ranges (for fun-filled patterns, try S'nack by S'well), and things like chilli con carne or curry go down really well the following day. The reason we paid a fortune for school dinners for so long is because I worried they wouldn't have something warm in their bellies during the winter. We could have saved a fortune and our kids would have eaten better had we worked this out sooner.

REUSABLE POUCHES AND SNACK BAGS

Firstly, any product that is reusable is a bonus when it comes to kids and food. 'Disposable' sounds great but, when you think of the sheer volume of stuff that kids go through, it's ideal to have something they can love and we can reuse. Reusable pouches and 'snack packs', such as the ones from DoddleBags above, are a-plenty, and it's not just good for the environment but you can often find them in themes that your kids will enjoy. Miraculously, they become more intrigued in what is inside AND they save you a fortune in the long run. Fill up a pouch with your own yogurt, fill up a snack bag with your own slices of fruit you know they will eat and voila, happy kiddo.

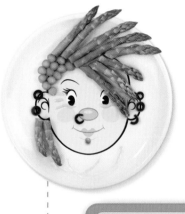

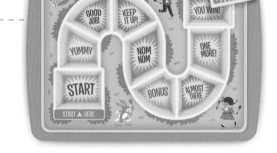

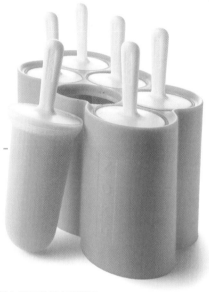

ICE LOLLY MAKERS

Getting your kids to eat ice lollies is of course really easy, so it's one of the sneaky ways I get fruit into Edith. I purée fruit with something like yogurt or her favourite juice and then freeze it. One of the best things I ever bought for the family was the Zoku Pop Maker. It freezes the lollies within minutes and, as long as I keep it in the freezer, I can just keep making fruity goodness lollies. Mwah ha ha!

THE SANDWICH CUTTER

You might think you're going to be wasteful with this one, but actually you're not. If your kids don't like crusts, there are loads of sandwich cutters that will remove the crust and turn the rest of your sandwich into whatever fun and funky shape you have purchased. Lunch Punch are probably the best ones I have found, but you can find a huge variety online.

DIVIDED PLATES

I always thought that divider plates were for toddlers but they are really good for picky eaters too. I'm a fan of a brand called Constructive Eating, who have been making fun divider and cutlery sets for years. I also recommend Fred & Friends' Dinner Winner game plates and Food Face plates. We were raised to believe that we must never play with our food, but in all honesty, who cares if they are pretending their fork is a digger and their knife is a fluttery fairy, if it means they eat the food you cooked?!

Simple chicken curry

(INSPIRED BY TAMING TWINS' ORIGINAL RECIPE)

As I've said before, I'm a big fan of recipes that are created by bloggers because often these people aren't chefs or qualified cooks but people like you and me who have trialled their recipes over and over with their own children and families. One of my favourite recipes is by a lovely blogger called Sarah who runs the website Taming Twins. It was the inspiration for the recipe that I do in my pressure cooker at least two or three times a month and it's my go-to for post after-school club meals. I also LOVE to change it up and play around with it. Serves 6

INGREDIENTS

3–4 chicken breasts or thighs
1 large onion, finely chopped
1 teaspoon garam masala
2 tablespoons mild curry powder
1 tablespoon ginger paste
2 tablespoons garlic paste
2 tablespoons mango chutney
1 x 400ml tin coconut milk
100g red lentils
1 large carrot, grated
salt and freshly ground black pepper

1. Place the chicken, onion, garam masala, curry powder, ginger and garlic in the pressure cooker on 'browning' mode and fry, stirring, for 3 minutes.

2. Add the rest of the ingredients and stir to combine. Attach the lid, set to 'meat' mode and cook for 20 minutes.

3. After 20 minutes, release the pressure. (This varies with each pressure cooker, but for mine I release the valve and then step back – the steam is crazy! Just mind your hands!) Take the chicken out and shred into a bowl.

4. Stir the chicken back into the curry and serve with rice and naan.

PLAY AROUND WITH THE INGREDIENTS
The best thing about this recipe is that it's so adaptable - try adding different fruit and veg, maybe something like dried apricots or some chickpeas. Play around with it to find your ideal speedy chicken curry!

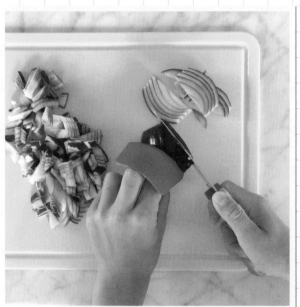

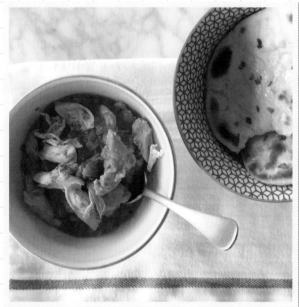

NO PRESSURE COOKER?
NO PROBLEM!

Place your chicken, onion, garam masala, curry powder, ginger and garlic in a deep casserole dish or heavy based saucepan that is oven safe – if you don't have one then use a frying pan to brown your ingredients for 5 minutes then transfer to a casserole dish. Add in the remaining ingredients, cover and cook for 90 minutes at 180°C/gas mark 4. Take out of the oven, shred the chicken and add back to the sauce before serving.

Cooking with kids

I think cooking with children is something that splits people into two camps. You're either like me and you quite enjoy it. You can just about cope with the mess and suppress the urge to say, 'Oh just give it here, I could have done it a million times over by now.' OR it's your nightmare and you hate it with the fiery passion of hell. In case you're curious, the latter is how I feel about crafting with children and explains why there is no chapter on weird and wonderful crafts that you can make with your kids in this book...

Regardless of which camp you fall into, there are so many ways you can make cooking with your kids a bit less painful. From the teeny tiny stage where they can just about hold a wooden spoon and 'help' or the tween stage where you are basically just supervising them and offering the use of your car should they need to get to A&E for a finger re-attachment. It's good for their mental and physical development and, ultimately, they have to learn some day because absolutely no one appreciates the roommate at uni who can't work out how to open a can of beans and who explodes the microwave.

Get organised

If I can impart one piece of advice throughout the entirety of this book, it's that getting organised BEFORE you involve your children is an essential part of any task. Before you suggest to them that you cook or bake together, get the things that you need out and ready.

I usually take 10 minutes to have a quick coffee and think about what we might need, read the recipe we're following and get everything out of the cupboards so I'm not leaving them to their own devices at any time. If you have one, it's also really useful to bake along with a device that supports Amazon Alexa, Google Home, etc., as it reads out a recipe so you're not checking what is next all the time.

MUM TIP: Keep all your mixers switched off at the socket until the second you need them. My kids will ALWAYS flick on the mixer the second I turn away, regardless of whether it is full or empty, so I've learnt to switch it off at the socket, and then every time they flick it on or off, it's just useless.

ONION TIP

I remember the first time Toby ever prepared dinner with me. He started to chop an onion, only to have the usual eye-watering reaction. Of course, this put him off chopping with me for ages. To avoid it, whether it's you or the kids, place your onions in the fridge as it calms down their pungency. You should be able to chop even the strongest without your eyes reacting.

MUM'S BAKING/COOKING CHECKLIST:

All ingredients
Measuring cups
Mixers/electric whisks
Utensils – whisks, mixing brushes, knives, rolling pins, etc.
Necessary pans and tins (I usually pre-line)
Tea towels – one for hands, one or two for inevitable mess
Bowls (I always have an extra one for eggs to be cracked into)
First aid kit fairly close to hand or at least an idea of where it is. Toby once grated all the way down his hand while grating cheese for a lasagne, so even when you think there is no way they will hurt themselves, the chances are they might. It's not the end of the world, and easier to cope with if you can sort any incidents quickly.
Medicinal booze of choice in your coffee cup for the eye-twitching moments.

Baking bread with kids

I never thought that baking bread was something I would do with my kids, but we got a taste for it during the coronavirus lockdown. It is time consuming but so worth it when you are dunking your bread into homemade soup or gravy. Not to mention the fact that it is SO much more economical than buying loaves from the supermarket.

500g strong bread flour, plus extra for dusting
2 teaspoons salt
7g fast-acting yeast (this is 1 sachet or 1 teaspoon)
3 tablespoons oil (I use sunflower but you can use olive oil too)
300ml water

1. In a large bowl, mix together your bread flour, salt and yeast. Make a well in the centre (always fun for the little ones to do) and then add your oil and water. Mix the ingredients well until all the flour is gone from around the edges. You can add a little bit more water if the mixture is too dry, but no more than 1–2 tablespoons.

2. Tip the dough out onto a well-floured surface and knead for 10 minutes until smooth. This is another great chance to get the kids involved – mine love beating the dough into various shapes.

3. Once you have a nice smooth dough, place it in a large, well-oiled bowl and cover the dough with a damp cloth so the top doesn't dry out. Set aside in a warm place for an hour or until it has doubled in size.

4. Now for the bit that is everyone's favourite – the knocking back, when you punch the dough to knock the air out. The boys thought this was hilarious and would always argue over who was to have the honour of doing it first.

5. Tip the dough out and knead again for 5 minutes. You shouldn't need to flour the surface for this bit. Shape the dough into a loaf shape (or whatever you like!) and place on a greased baking tray, then cover once again with a damp cloth and set aside for another hour or until it doubles in size.

7. Preheat your oven to 200°C/gas mark 6 and, with a sharp knife, cut across the dough in diagonal stripes, no more than 1cm deep.

8. Finally, bake for 25-30 minutes until golden and you hear a nice hollow sound when you tap the underneath of the dough. Allow to cool slightly but try eating it warm because it is GLORIOUS with lots of melting butter. NOM.

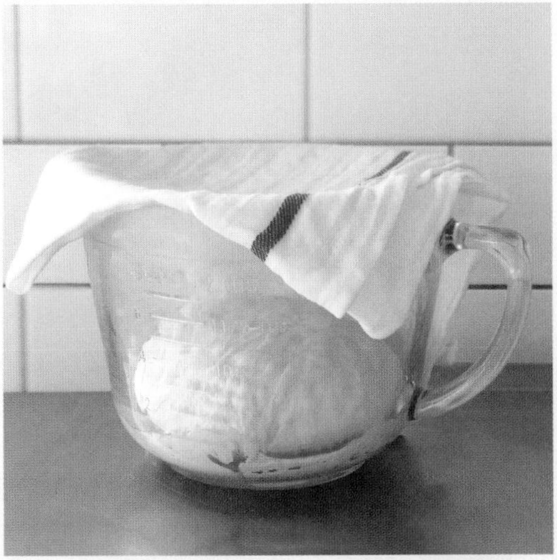

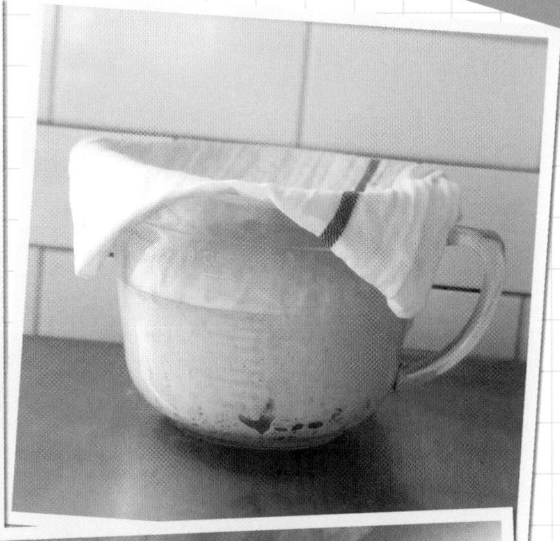

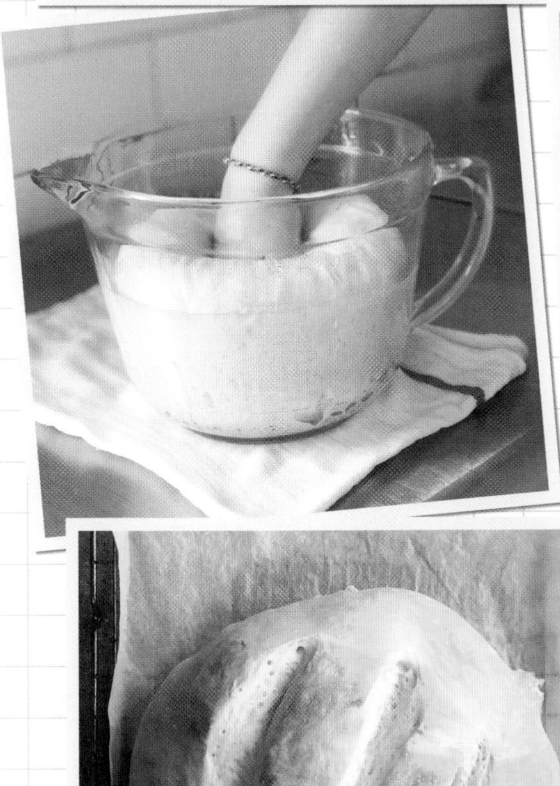

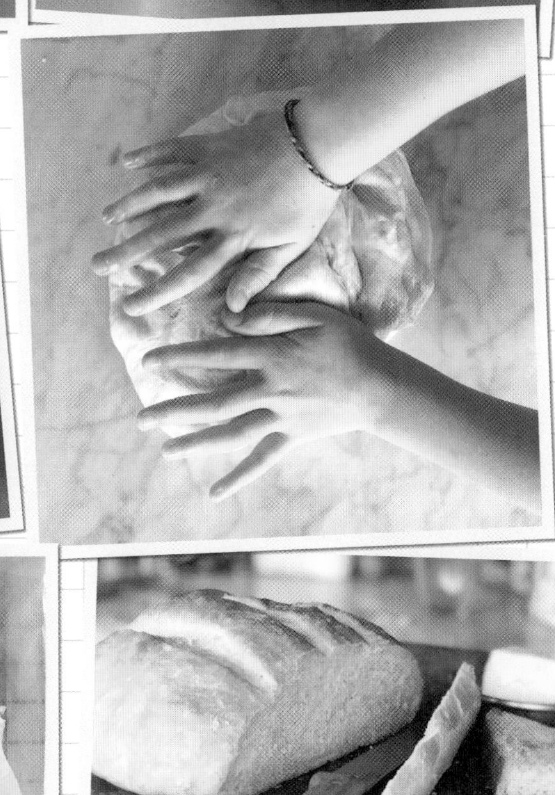

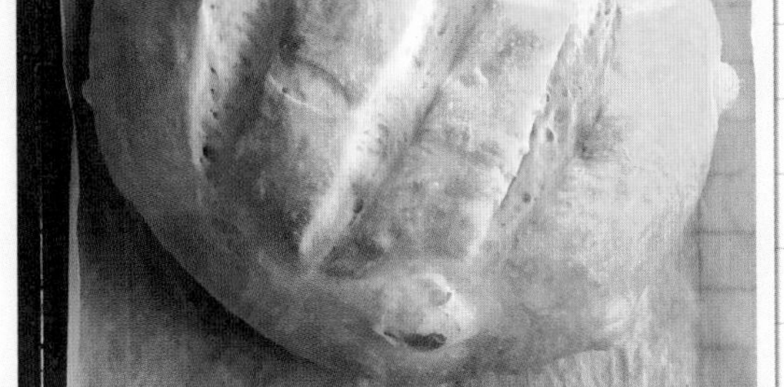

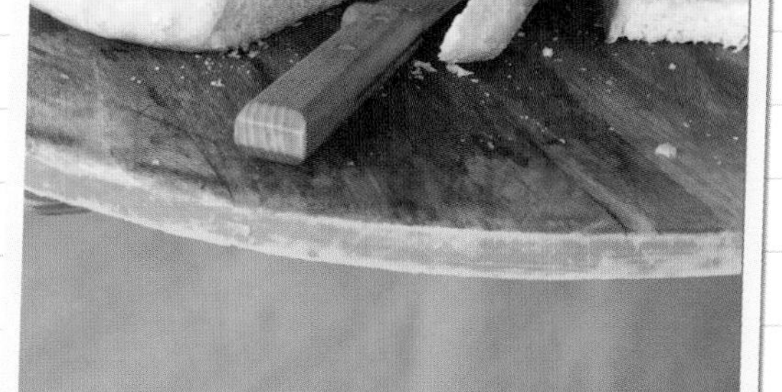

Simple brownies

Brownies are one of the easiest (and tastiest) things to make with your kids and this is my absolute favourite recipe – amazingly chewy and gooey. I've put the recipe in cups for two reasons, firstly because I actually really love working with the American measuring system of cups – it's just SO easy. Secondly, because cups are easier for little hands, measuring the mixture out this way can make things a lot less painful. It's also a good opportunity to reinforce home learning with fractions and numbers.

INGREDIENTS

1 cup (200g) granulated sugar
¼ cup (50g) soft brown sugar
75g unsalted butter, melted
3 eggs
¾ cup (75g) cocoa powder
⅓ cup (80ml) sunflower oil
pinch of salt
½ cup (64g) plain flour
1 tablespoon cornflour
150g white chocolate, broken into chunks
150g milk chocolate, broken into chunks
icing sugar, for dusting (optional)

1. Preheat your oven to 200°C/gas mark 6. Grease and line a 20cm square cake tin with greaseproof paper.

2. In a microwave-proof bowl, mix together the sugars and butter, then microwave on a medium heat for 1 minute and stir together.

3. Whisk the eggs into the butter and sugar mixture and add the oil. Stir in the cocoa powder, salt and flours.

4. Fold in the chocolates, keeping them in quite sizeable chunks so that you get pockets of melted chocolate in the brownies.

5. Tip the brownie mixture into the prepared tin and bake in the oven for 30 minutes.

6. Allow to cool on a cooling rack inside the greaseproof paper but do not cool completely – eat while still warm!

7. As a finishing touch, dust with icing sugar or serve as they are.

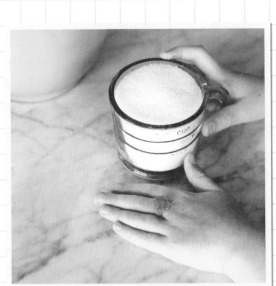
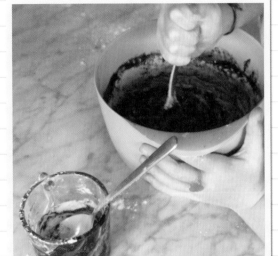
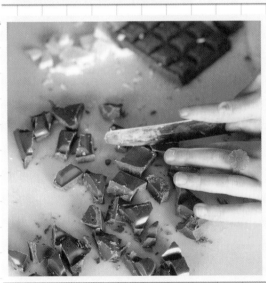
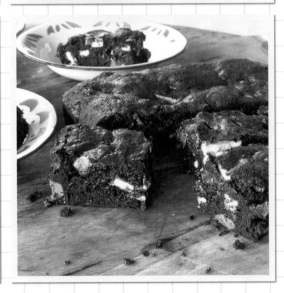

A little chef's tools

I've always been a big believer in not purchasing lots of things for the kids to use in the kitchen because they can use our things just as easily and I often think it's merely a nifty way to get parents to spend more. That being said, there are a few things that are worth investing in if you're planning on having regular cooking and baking sessions with your children.

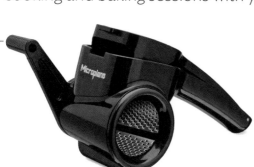

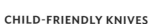

ROTARY GRATER

Many a kitchen cut and scrape in our family has come from the grater: the kids are grating like the clappers, marvelling at the mound of cheese filling up the middle and then BAM they grate their knuckles and I'm left sorting through grated cheese to check we're not going vaguely cannibal for dinner, while also administering a cold compress. Rotary graters like this one from Microplane eliminate that risk, especially for younger kids, and they're a fun bit of kit to use. Oxo do a Seal and Store Rotary Grater that you can use to grate and then store whatever you grated in the fridge.

CHILD-FRIENDLY KNIVES

Now, I include this because I know it is a huge barrier for a lot of people when it comes to letting children cook. I'll level with you – we don't use child-friendly knives. My kids use the same knives I do, heavily supervised. I think it's important to teach them from a young age that knives need to be handled properly. If it is something that you are anxious about, there are loads of child-friendly knives. There are ones made out of nylon that are not completely childproof, so a bit like the kid scissors you have in schools, but I've never found one that can cut a carrot or broccoli. I like Opinel's Le Petit Chef knives, which are still sharp, but they're small and come with a finger guard and a place for that little supporting finger. I also recommend using an egg slicer if you have a really tiny one cooking with you, as they're great for cutting soft things.

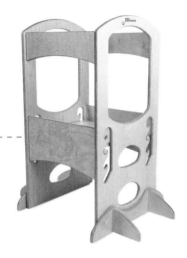

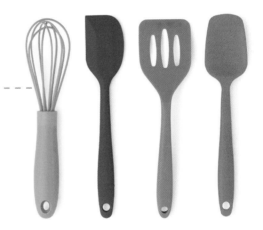

THE LEARNING TOWER

There are so many versions of this but, when Reuben was little, we bought the original Learning Tower from Little Partners for him to stand in so he could cook with me and it was the best investment for the kitchen we ever made. The concept is simple: it elevates the child in a safe way and allows them to stand secure and steady so they can't slip or fall when you are cooking. You can then easily move about the kitchen, grabbing the things you need, without panicking about hearing that dreaded BANG and scream when they have toppled off the stool. Is it a necessity? Absolutely not. We re-homed ours when we were renovating and Edith bakes/cooks without one, but she has fallen off stools and I really do miss it. I highly recommend the Little Partners one (you can buy nifty covers for it too that turn it into a shop and other things so it can have more uses).

UTENSILS

Essential? No. Cute? You betcha. As I said above, they often aren't necessary, but if you have a child who really loves cooking or baking, having their own equipment, like these colourful utensils from Lakeland, can feel really special. We all remember the first time we moved out of home and started shopping for our own kitchen stuff – it feels so grown up – and for kids that is a huge thing. Edith insists on using her own bright pink, cake-emblazoned spatula, and it's a running joke in Adam's family that, as a teen, he put 'omelette pan' on his Christmas wish list because he wanted to have some of his own pans! Independence is a good thing where cooking is concerned.

Lemon slices

Ridiculously easy and simple to make, these are something that my boys can happily make without me now – though they rarely make it through without wanting to throttle one another and are usually covered in mixture fairly quickly. It's a great way to break away from cups and go for metric measurements, without being too much for tiny ones.

INGREDIENTS

110g unsalted butter
110g caster sugar
2 eggs
110g plain flour
1 teaspoon baking powder
zest of 1 lemon
2–3 drops lemon essence
   (I prefer this over lemon juice)
2 tablespoons icing sugar

1. Preheat the oven to 200°C/gas mark 6. Grease and line a 20cm square cake tin with greaseproof paper.

2. In a bowl, cream the butter and sugar until pale and fluffy.

3. Add the eggs along with a tablespoon of the flour (it will help to stop the mixture splitting), and mix together.

4. Add the remaining flour, baking powder, lemon zest and lemon essence and stir to combine.

5. Pour the cake batter into the prepared tin and bake for 15–20 minutes or until a skewer inserted into the middle comes out clean.

6. Transfer to a cooling rack and, when cool, cut into slices – we usually do a similar size and style to Kipling cakes.

7. Place the icing sugar in a bowl and mix with a little water. For this part, I usually fill up an old (clean) medicine syringe and let the kids squirt in a bit of water at a time – they think it's great fun! Once the icing is at 'drizzle' consistency, simply flick it back and forth over your cake slices. If you feel fancy, you can add lemon juice or essence to the icing, or even some yellow food colouring. Whatever tickles your pickle!

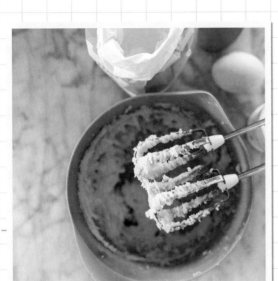

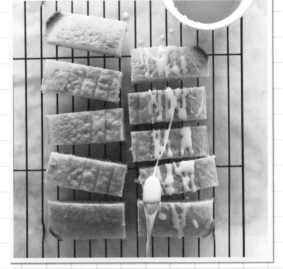

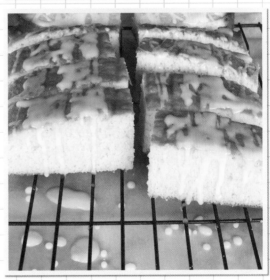

PYO (pick your own)

Every year, around later summer time, I decide that I would like to do pick your own (PYO) with the kids, and not just for the Instagram pictures (don't look at me like that). No, I want to do it for two reasons. Firstly, it entertains us for a few hours and gets us out of the house, and we're talking minimum four-and-a-half hours if I go to one of those fabulous farm shop places that offers PYO and has a glorious, overpriced café attached.

The second reason is absolutely the one that sways me more: **Rum Pot**. If you haven't heard of a rum pot, then I'm going to introduce you to it (page 48), because it is the holy grail of PYO. We have been gifting it to family and friends for the last four or five years (and mainly saving it to drink ourselves). You pick your own fruit across the seasons and then, for every layer of fruit that you add to a Kilner jar or container of some fashion, you add a layer of sugar and coat it in alcohol until it's completely full of fruits, booze and sugar. It makes one hell of a tipple, usually ready *just* in time for Christmas. It's also perfection drizzled over ice cream because it's so syrupy (thanks to months and months of sugary fermentation).

RUM POT
An easy, simple alcoholic drink that is fun for little hands to help make because they can pick the fruit, pour the sugar and you can add the booze. You can even do it with water if you aren't comfortable with alcohol, though it doesn't taste as good.

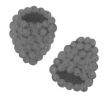

So, here are the all-important PYO fruits for our rum pot. The season for picking will depend on where you live in the world – what other fruits could you add?

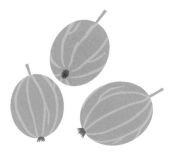

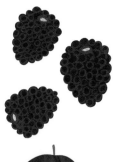

STRAWBERRIES

RASPBERRIES

GOOSEBERRIES

CURRANTS

BLUEBERRIES

BLACKBERRIES

PLUMS

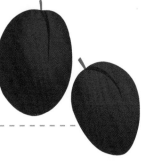

WHY PICK YOUR OWN WHEN YOU CAN GRAB IT IN THE SUPERMARKET?

PYO is undoubtably more expensive, to be totally honest with you. The last time we went, we spent so much on strawberries and raspberries that Adam exclaimed at the checkout, 'Are they laced with gold dust?!' Of course, it was an extortionate amount to spend on a couple of punnets and yet we did spend over three hours in the fields and then another hour and a half in the café while the kids played happily. We had an almost full day out for the price of a few punnets and some coffee and cake and even brought something home, so I'd call that a bargain.

The other side of the coin is that you can't lose with the quality of farm-fresh fruit. It simply tastes better than anything from a supermarket. It's fresher, it's usually

laced with far fewer chemicals and it's completely ripe. I also think, if I'm going to be steeping it to make Christmas gifts in the boozy format or jam, it's worth having the very best I can get my mittens on to.

And again, the aforementioned entertainment factor for you and the children is unbeatable. It really can be fun and most PYO farms encourage you to bring a picnic as they want you to stick around and pick more fruit (just make sure you don't eat too much as you go – it's accepted that you'll taste what you're picking and try stopping those kids! – but it's not fair to the farms to be excessive as PYO is done on weight). You can usually get some kind of discount too if you become a regular. Always ask if they have a loyalty scheme.

Rum pot

Rum pot is one of my favourite things to make with the kids. A lovely woman from my Instagram community suggested it to me after I made some Pumpkin vodka one Halloween. Her advice: try it drizzled over ice cream!

INGREDIENTS

1 litre Kilner jar

any fruits you have picked
  (you want enough of each to
  create a good two-finger layer
  in the jar that you use.
  I personally love strawberries,
  raspberries, blueberries,
  blackberries and plums, but
  it really can be any fruit of your
  choice. For large fruit, chop
  into smaller pieces so you
  can cram more in.

caster sugar – for every layer
  you will need 115g sugar

cheap white rum
  (it's more likely to take on
  the flavour)

1. Make sure that your jar is very clean, ideally sterilised. Add your first layer of fruit (probably strawberries as they will be the first in season) and cover with a layer of sugar. Pour in the rum to just above the fruit and sugar, then seal the jar and leave in a cool, dark location until you are ready to add your next layer. DO NOT SHAKE.

2. When you are ready for the next layer of fruit, repeat the same process, and seal again. Keep adding your PYO fruit until you have a full jar. With each layer, you will notice that the previous fruit has 'melted' down, thus making more room.

3. When you add your final layer of fruit and sugar, seal and leave for a minimum of two weeks.

4. When you're ready, strain the mixture using a fine sieve and voila! Rum pot all round.

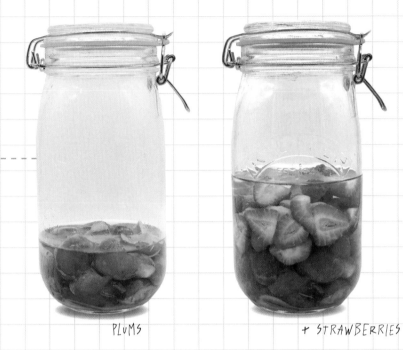
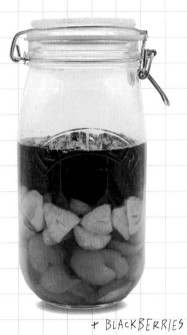

PLUMS

+ STRAWBERRIES

+ BLACKBERRIES

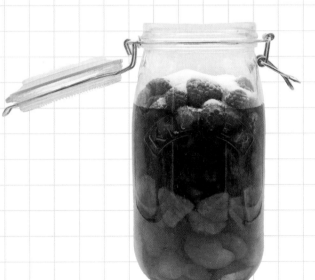
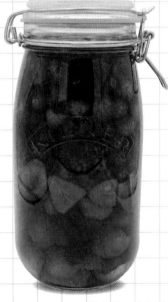

+ RASPBERRIES

+ BLACK CURRANTS

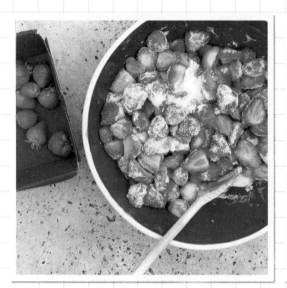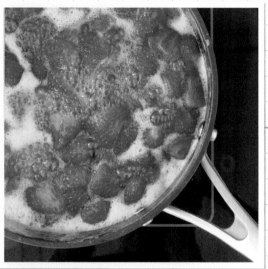
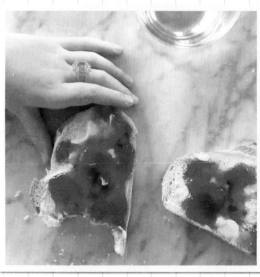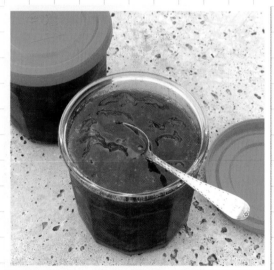

Simple strawberry and vanilla jam

Jam is a great thing to make with children as they are always more accepting of things they have helped to make, and it's also a great way to teach them caution in the kitchen, but be really careful – hot sugar burns are the worst!

INGREDIENTS

1kg PYO strawberries

750g jam sugar

1 teaspoon vanilla extract (or 2 vanilla pods)

Juice of 1 lemon

1. Wipe your strawberries clean. They don't need rinsing because they will end up absorbing water.

2. Toss the strawberries in the sugar and leave overnight or, if you have children who want to get going, you can do this in the morning and then finish the recipe in the afternoon. A minimum of 4 hours is needed for those strawberries to absorb some of the sugar.

3. Place the fruit in a saucepan over a low heat and add the lemon juice and vanilla extract or pods. Gently increase the heat until all of the sugar has dissolved.

4. Bring to the boil and cook for 10 minutes. I don't actually have a thermometer to check my jam (if you do, you want to reach 105°C) so I use the 'saucer method'. If I place a teaspoon of jam on a cold saucer (pop one in the fridge before you try) and it sets and wrinkles when I push my finger against it, it's done. If it's still runny, it's not.

5. Set aside for 15 minutes, then take the vanilla pods out if you used them and scrape off any scum on the top.

6. Before you place the jam in jars, warm them up. Add some slightly cooled boiled water to the empty jar and then pour away. Because the sugar is so hot, this stops the jar shattering when you add the jam.

7. Fill the jars with jam and place a wax disc on the top before screwing on the lid – this stops mildew. You can store it for up to a year but refrigerate once it has been opened.

Gifting homemade treats

I've talked a lot about how we gift the things we make from our hand-picked fruit (pages 48-51). It's such a fun thing to do, not to mention ridiculously popular with the grandparents, and cheaper than buying gifts for everyone that they might not even appreciate or like.

In recent years, we've embellished the idea and started to make Christmas hampers for the older members of our family. We fill them with all sorts of tasty treats that the kids and I have made together, as well as some really lovely foods from the local deli. Food is something that unites the vast majority of adults and, when it comes to homemade gifts from your little ones, there is rarely a faster way to a grandparent's heart.

I love to make a nice big hamper. I break it down over a series of weekends and 'free time' during November and December (obviously foodie things need to be nearer the time) and it feels like a lovely lead-up to the holidays. I work on a 'buy and make' basis, so we will perhaps buy a nice selection of deli cheese and a small gift (usually bed socks or a candle) and put them in the hamper, surrounded by things the kids have spent rainy weekends making. It fills up very easily and doesn't stress me out half as much as trying to source last-minute presents while simultaneously trying to meet deadlines and attend and prep for the billion social events that each of my kids seems to spring upon me at the end of every year.

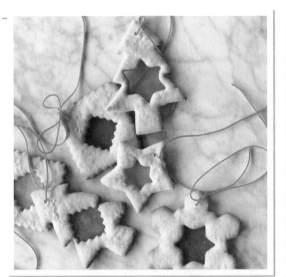

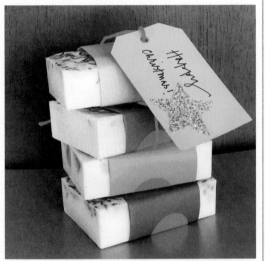

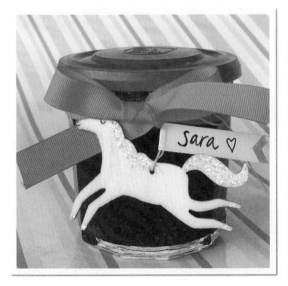

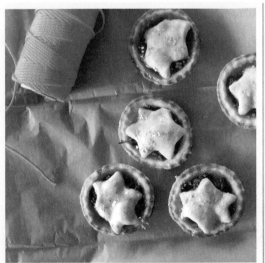

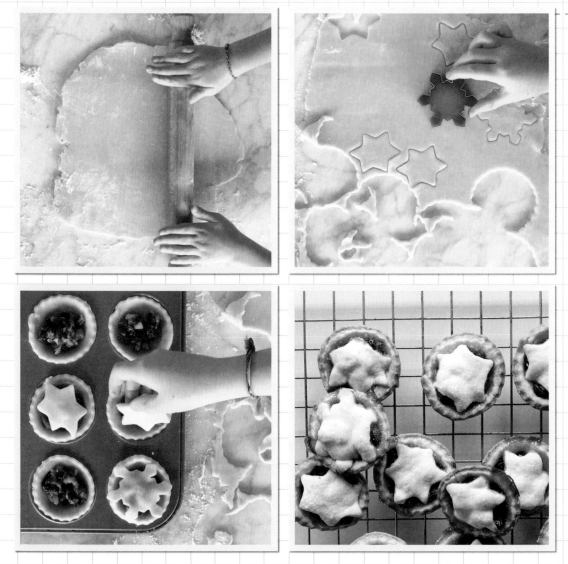

Easy cheat's mince pies

Mince pies are one of my favourite things about the run up to Christmas. They are remarkably easy to make, scent your house better than a candle and make you want to flounce around the kitchen singing 'All I want for Christmas' like you're Mariah. **Makes approx. 12**

FOR THE FILLING:
Jar of pre-made mince pie filling
1–2 tablespoons orange zest
1–2 tablespoons lemon zest
handful of finely chopped
    dried apricots
handful of finely chopped
    glacé cherries
1 apple (skin on), grated
2–3 tablespoons Cointreau
    (optional, depends on whether
    the recipient wants to share with
    children or not. You can sub with
    any brandy, rum or whisky)

FOR THE PASTRY:
225g plain flour
150g cold butter, diced
1 egg, beaten
75g icing sugar

1. First make the pastry. Sift the flour into a large bowl and mix through the diced butter. Rub both together with your fingertips until the mixture is the consistency of fine breadcrumbs. Mix in the egg and sugar. At this point, it may seem more like a paste than a workable pastry – don't panic, this is normal. Wrap in clingfilm and store in the fridge for at least 1 hour.

2. To make the filling, mix all of the ingredients together in a bowl and inhale deeeeeply so as to enjoy those wonderful Christmassy smells. Set aside to marinate for a minimum of 1 hour, better still overnight.

3. Preheat your oven to 180°C/gas mark 4.

4. When you come to roll out the pastry, work quickly as otherwise it will revert to a paste-like consistency. Have a circle cutter (about 10cm) and star cutter to hand and lightly grease a 12-hole tart tin/muffin tin.

5. On a well-floured surface, roll the pastry out to 3mm thick. Using the circle cutter, cut out 12 bases and place in your tart/muffin tin.

6. Spoon a teaspoon of mixture (a little bit more if you feel it needs it) onto the middle of each base. Cut out the remaining pastry into star shapes (circles if you don't feel fancy), and place on top.

7. Bake the pies in the oven for 12 minutes or until you see blissfully golden pastry. Set aside and allow to cool before popping in a little gift cake box and tying with ribbons. Alternatively, just gift them to yourself with a glass of eggnog. The mince pies will usually keep for up to 7 days if stored in a sealed container in a cool, dry place.

So, what should

the foodie

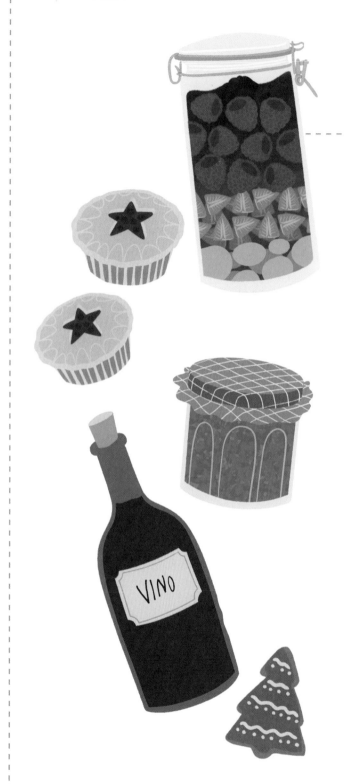

Rum Pot page 48

Homemade alcohol liqueurs

Favourite alcoholic drink

Swanky mixers

Homemade (or not) jam

Mince pies page 55

Brownies page 40

Christmas cake

Sweet treats – homemade or shop-bought (highly recommend ordering from bettys.co.uk for the fancy wow factor)

Fudge (fudgekitchen.co.uk if you don't have the time or inclination to make it)

Nice oils & balsamic or flavoured vinegars

Bread (buy last-minute or bake)

Biscuits

Meats and cheese (last-minute buy!)

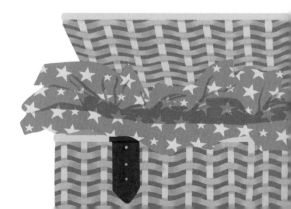

go in my hamper?

a little gift

A DVD

A pair of bed socks

A Christmas decoration

A Christmas tree ornament

Perfume

Bubble bath

Beauty products, like hand scrub

(very easy to make)

Bath bomb (homemade)

Homemade soap

(easier than you think to make, page 60)

Kids' artworks

Candle

Spacemasks

(deliciously relaxing sleep masks spacemasks.com)

Diary or stationery

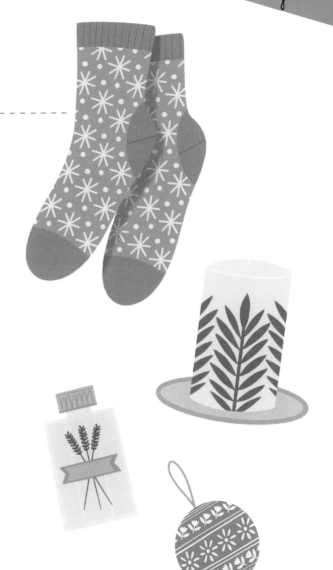

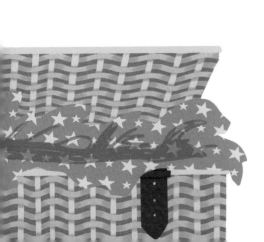

Stained glass biscuits

These are some of the cutest things I've ever made with my kids. They are really simple and easy to make with that wow factor that makes a perfect addition to any hamper. They are lovely little decorations to pop on the Christmas tree too. **Makes approx. 30 biscuits**

INGREDIENTS

1 cup (225g) butter
1 ¼ cups (280g) caster sugar
2 eggs, plus 2 yolks
3 cups (385g) plain flour
¾ teaspoon baking powder
¾ teaspoon salt
2 teaspoons vanilla extract
 (I recommend Nielsen-Massey pure vanilla extract for this)
1 bag (approx. 100g) hard-boiled sweets

MUM TIP: Skewer a tiny hole into the top of the biscuit, and once it's cooked, you can thread some ribbon through to make it into a hanging decoration.

1. Preheat the oven to 180°C/gas mark 4.

2. In a large bowl, cream together the butter and sugar until pale, light and fluffy. Add 2 eggs and a spoonful of the flour to stop the mixture splitting. Add the 2 egg yolks and the remaining flour, the baking powder, salt and vanilla extract and mix until you have a smooth, crumbly biscuit dough. Pop the dough in the fridge for 15 minutes.

3. Take the chilled dough and roll out onto a floured surface to 8–10mm thick, then cut into shapes of your choice. Make sure your cutters are fairly large as you then need to cut out a space in the middle of each biscuit to contain the 'stained glass'. You can use a small star cutter to cut a star shape inside a large star, or cut a circle or any shape you fancy.

4. Arrange the biscuits on a baking tray lined with baking paper and place in the oven for 8-10 minutes.

5. Meanwhile, group your hard-boiled sweets into colours, place in a bag or between two sheets of parchment paper and bash with a rolling pin until crushed (my kids love that bit!).

6. Take the biscuits out of the oven and DO NOT move them. Instead, sprinkle the crushed sweets inside the space in the centre of each biscuit, then pop them back in the oven for 3-4 minutes.

7. The sweets should have melted and created a lovely coloured glass effect. Allow the biscuits to cool on the tray or they will break. Voila!

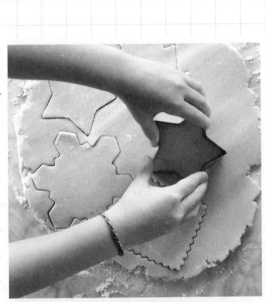
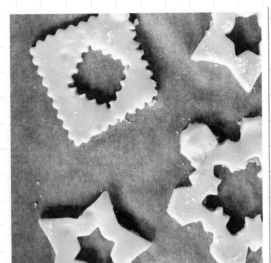
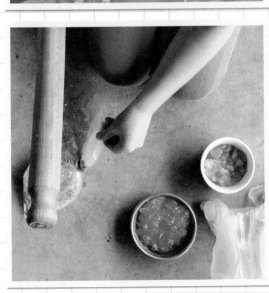
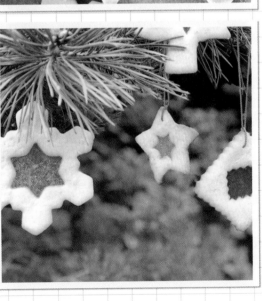

You can also **MAKE YOUR OWN DRIED FLOWER PETALS** for your soap using this clever little microwave hack! Buy flowers from the supermarket or find some you are allowed to pick in the wild. Separate the petals and place them on a sheet of kitchen paper on a microwave-safe plate. Microwave on the high setting for 1 minute, then add 30 second blasts until the petals are crisp.

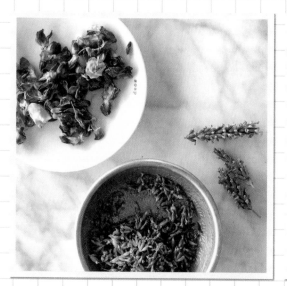

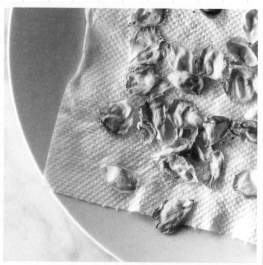

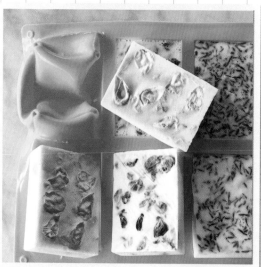

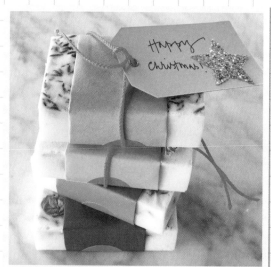

Homemade soap

Soap is pretty universal – we all need to use it, so it makes a lovely little addition to a hamper. We've made a variety of soaps over the years using all manner of moulds that I had in the baking cupboard for cakes and chocolates, even using plastic food-storage containers to create a big slab that we cut into rectangles for a more traditional soap. This will make roughly 4 larger rectangular bars of soap, but it really depends on what shape you're going for!

YOU WILL NEED

silicone soap moulds (you can buy these online), or you can use cake or chocolate moulds or a plastic food container

500g shea butter soap base (opaque or white are my fave – you can buy big tubs online)

Essential oil/s of your choice (Rose is classic but if you'd like something more refreshing, try a citrus. Don't be afraid to mix scents too – geranium and lemon are lovely together. The soaps opposite use rose, geranium and lavender oils)

Rose petals or lavender, as desired (the soaps opposite also use wisteria petals)

1. Place the soap base in a microwave-proof bowl and melt slowly in the microwave. I would recommend 30–60 second blasts on a medium-high heat depending on your microwave to ensure it doesn't overheat. If it does over heat it's likely to become clumpy and impossible to use.

2. Add a few drops of essential oils to the mixture, usually 5–6 drops will do it, and give it a good stir. Add your petals or decoration if you have chosen to use it – it's really up to you whether you want to stir it in or sit it on top!

3. Pour the liquid soap into the mould and set in the fridge overnight.

4. Tie the bar of soap with string or ribbon and add a label and you have a beautifully natural, lovely-smelling homemade gift.

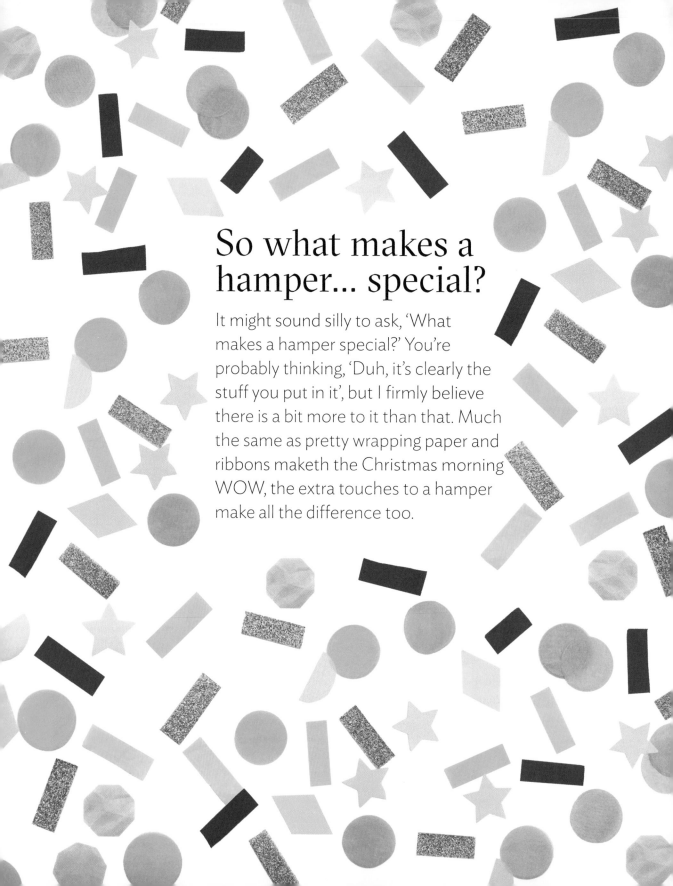

So what makes a hamper... special?

It might sound silly to ask, 'What makes a hamper special?' You're probably thinking, 'Duh, it's clearly the stuff you put in it', but I firmly believe there is a bit more to it than that. Much the same as pretty wrapping paper and ribbons maketh the Christmas morning WOW, the extra touches to a hamper make all the difference too.

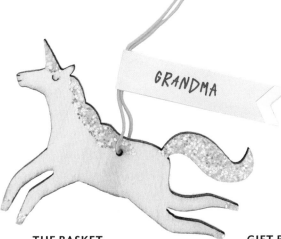

GRANDMA

THE BASKET

For a really special hamper, I start off with a wicker basket – these are so easy to find these days and come in different shapes and sizes and with lids and without. A hamper with a lid is usually more pricey and I find the lid can be a pain if you're filling it with large bottles or Kilner jars, so bear that in mind.

TISSUE PAPER

People underestimate the power of tissue paper, in my opinion, and it's a great way to make any hamper a little more luxurious. It comes in a huge variety of colours and is also eco-friendly as it's made from recycled materials, so you can give your hamper a lovely colourful lining and an instant bit of flare (and if someone gifts you a hamper, save the paper because one day you might want to use it yourself!).

CONFETTI & SPARKLES

This is a bit of a controversial one as confetti and sparkles need to be chosen carefully. You can find some amazing eco-friendly options if you do want to add this as a final finishing touch!

GIFT BOXES FOR SWEET TREATS

Nothing kills the mood of 'I spent time making this' as quickly as a Tupperware box or, worse still, a takeaway carton. With food, it's always worth thinking about presentation and there are loads of gift boxes and bags out there, even in supermarkets now. If you want to go the extra mile, your best bet is a shop like Lakeland or Hobbycraft. You can also find downloadable templates online from places like Canon Creative Park.

RIBBONS & GIFT TAGS

Not just for wrapping around gifts under the tree, a little tie of ribbon can take a box of homemade cookies in a plain box from 'I didn't have enough time or money this year to buy a fancy gift' to 'I put a lot of thought into this and is way better than anything I could have bought'. Ribbon is a great way to tie up a hamper if you chose one with a lid and don't forget to add gift tags as the effect is the same. You can make them, print them, buy them – the unicorn tag here is from Meri Meri – whatever works for you! I guess it's a psychology thing but it reiterates we made this especially for you and, well, it means something.

notes

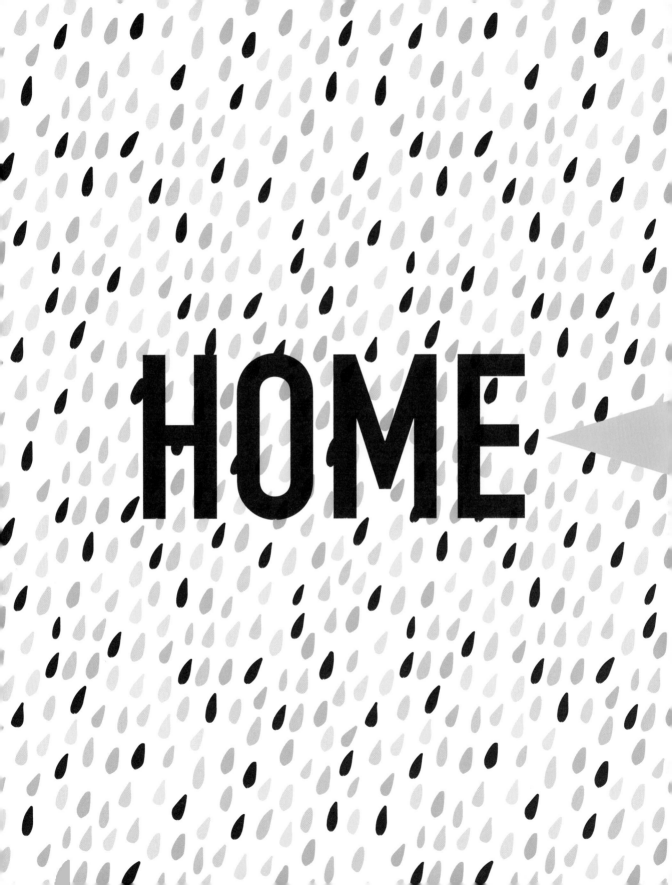

When I was a little girl, I used to spend countless hours creating 'homes' out of boxes. I'd carefully choose 'wallpaper', either that I had made using my felt tips or using a sheet from DIY shop 'tester' rolls. I'd cut rugs out of my mum's magazines and I'd use my Playmobil and Sylvanian furniture to create rooms in different spaces. I'd add stickers to the walls for 'artwork' or set up the dining table like one of the show homes we visited when we moved house when I was nine years old.

I loved playing house; it's such a fun memory of my childhood – apart from the slightly traumatising moment when I used my hamster as a house guest and he peed all over my carefully crafted shoebox living room and gave new meaning to the name 'Whizzer', which we'd given him.

However, my point is that I've always loved 'playing house', stamping my style onto rooms like Peppa Pig stamps in muddy puddles. For years, I dreamt about owning my own home and having the opportunity to style it how I wanted. Bless my 14-year-old self! However, eventually I did get a home of my own and, with a lot of saving and borrowing, enough to do some of the things I wanted to do. (Sadly, though, no heated pool with an LA-style waterfall and view that my Sims had, oh and without the household staff.) And then of course along came the realisation that this wasn't *just* my home to decorate and style as I liked but, in fact, **a home with small children, a husband who wanted to put his own stamp on things, pets, dirty football boots, school bags, paperwork, dead plants in vases... it was a real home, lived in and imperfect**. This was reality and it didn't look anything like the shoebox house of yesteryear (well, actually, maybe after Whizzer the hamster peed in it...).

Home really is where the heart is but sometimes your heart is limited by pesky things like budget, children and partners. Sometimes it's limited by reality. The good news is that nowadays there are so many wonderful, affordable ways to hack your home, and to create the space that works for everyone in the family and doesn't compromise any of the things that make it yours. You're never more than a few clicks away from a hack to upcycle or a way to get clean and tidy without spending hours slaving away. **In this next chapter I'm going to share with you everything I have learned about hacking my home, keeping my style and making life just that bit easier for myself.**

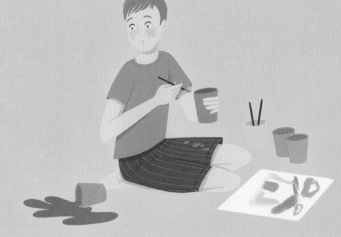

Keeping your style while keeping it real

I worked in children's retail at Mothercare for seven years, both before and after I became a mum. I was positioned in the home and travel department, so, if you asked me anything about toys or fashion I would look at you with a blank face and mutter something about finding someone to help you, but ask me which stair gate or cot was best for you and I was your girl.

When we become parents, we often stop thinking so much about our style and replace our preferences with 'what is best for the baby or children' or 'what will last with the children playing on it'. It's not necessarily a bad thing, but it often means that you end up with a home filled with interim items; a sofa in a colour you aren't really that keen on, or you put away all your beloved vases because you don't want them smashed.

My first Mum friend utterly dismissed this latter attitude in favour of keeping her style and her favourite things. She hadn't long decorated her home before she found out that she was expecting (on her wedding day) and so her attitude was very much 'nope, this baby will not change my home'. So, when it came to child-proofing her home, she just... didn't. We met at a baby group and a little bunch of us formed a lovely friendship while all on maternity leave. Every Wednesday, we would have a cake and coffee morning at each other's houses and her house had beautiful wooden floors and gorgeous glass ornaments and vases adorned all the window sills. However, at around the age of eleven to twelve months, our little ones had just worked out how to grab and pull whatever they could get their little mittens on.

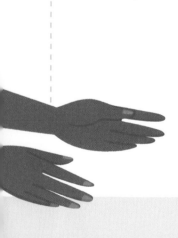

One day, one of the other mums (let's call her friend B) in the group (who was, admittedly, a very free-range mum and rarely used the word 'no') allowed her daughter to climb onto our friend's (friend A) window sill. She was standing chatting while holding her daughter's back and stopping her from falling as if it was the most normal thing in the world for your kid to be clambering near someone else's prized ornaments and vases. I remember, I was standing nearby, aware that Friend A seemed about ready to scream, 'Get your child away from my breakables!' and wondering how friend B could be so oblivious to her child getting precariously closer and closer to toppling a vase and smashing it on the wood below. Eventually, friend A tensely but politely asked if friend B would take her baby away from the window sill and you would have thought at this point that friend B would have twigged that it was a little rude to assume her beloved child could climb anywhere in anyone's home... but no. No, friend B lifted her daughter down and declared with a smile, 'Oh sorry, I didn't think it would be a problem. I mean, you're going to have to move them if you don't want them smashing anyway, aren't you? Bit silly to have them there with babies and toddlers in the house.' Regardless of whether you agree with this assessment, nothing feels quite

as uncomfortable as sitting between two friends who obviously have very different views on the way their kids are being raised. Friend A simply smiled and replied, 'Well actually no, we are going to teach our child not to climb around the house and she won't be allowed to touch things that she can break. Accidents might happen but she will learn that there are things that she can't touch, just like sharp things.' Needless to say, it was one of the last times we met together as a group. And I remember thinking that really my friend wasn't wrong. Sometimes there has to be a balance between what you want to have in your home and keeping your children safe.

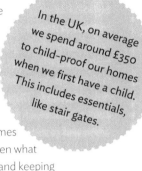

In the UK, on average we spend around £350 to child-proof our homes when we first have a child. This includes essentials, like stair gates.

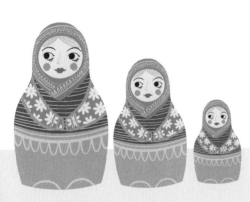

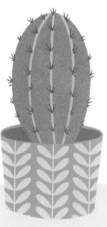

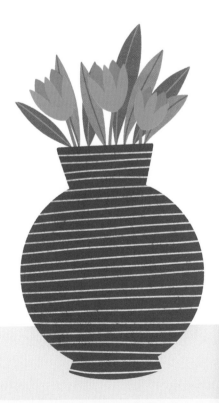

Letting go of child friendly

When we were remodelling the ground floor of our house, one of the things that we kept saying to the builders was that things needed to be 'child-friendly'. For example, the corners of the kitchen counters had to be rounded off to avoid any nasty bumps on little heads and all the flooring needed to be really heavy duty and tough. Then we went and painted the whole ground floor in white and pastels. Hmm.

Look, the concept of child-friendly is often one we take to the extreme and I don't believe it should have to mean a complete sacrifice of style so that our homes look like something from the Fun Factory in 1998. We can still have the things we love and we can still keep our kids safe.

So where do we go wrong?

'Wrong' sounds a bit harsh. It's more, where do we start to lose ourselves and completely change our style in our home because we have kids. 'That's too breakable, that's too dangly, that's just too expensive to potentially be damaged.' I never did this when I had pets but I guarantee you that my cats and dogs have damaged just as many delicate or expensive items as my children, possibly more. To put it another way, we still have expensive things – a TV, for instance, and we don't say, 'Hmm, maybe I should look at buying a smaller, less expensive one because my kiddo might accidentally break it'.

Our sofas are all velvet and I have lost count of the number of times that friends and family members told us not to buy them because they wouldn't be 'tough enough for the kids'. However, they haven't worn as badly as everyone expected them to. We have rules – the kids aren't allowed to eat on the sofas, for any spills we use a 'spill kit' that I bought when we got the sofas, and we put blankets down if someone is poorly.

We lose so much of ourselves when we become parents that I think it's important to remember to buy the things that we love. Take a leaf out of my friend's book – we don't have to change everything, we maybe just have to change the way we approach it. So what if it's breakable? So what if it's not made of plastic that is ultra-hardwearing? It's your home, too.

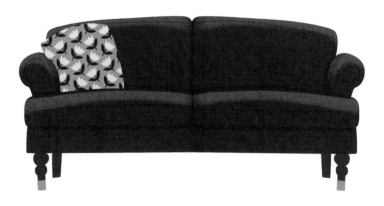

Creating shared and personal spaces

WHAT ARE THE ESSENTIALS OF CHILD-FRIENDLY?

When I worked in children's retail at Mothercare, they stocked a vast range of products that really are essential for your home if you have children. Stair gates, for example, or socket protectors to stop children from jabbing their fingers or objects into sockets and harming themselves. These kinds of things really are the essentials as they can directly impact a child's health and safety. Therefore, in my opinion, the debate boils down to child safety vs. child friendly.

We have been really firm since we renovated the ground floor as it's filled with things that we all love. I spent a lot of time thinking about the way that we live and what works for us as a family unit, but also unashamedly about myself and what I liked. Admittedly we were fortunate enough to be having a renovation, but when I look back I have always tried to create family/shared spaces and personal spaces beyond individual bedrooms. Reuben used to have a chair in the hallway where he could just go and sit quietly, watching his iPad and relaxing. The old living room housed both my office space and our family space, both co-existing in a slightly awkward yet workable space.

Having areas that are your own, even within a shared space, are absolutely essential as it's where you can create your own rules. These days, now I have an office to work in, all of my own, I love that it's preserved as a space for me. My children wouldn't ever feel shy about coming in to ask a question or have a chat but they also understand that this is MY space and they wouldn't bring in toys or play in there unless I gave them permission.

And it's the same for our children when they start to create their own spaces. It's incredibly hard as there's only so much to go around and a child can't always have a bedroom of their own and must share. Until my eldest turned seven, he shared a room with his younger brother, Toby, and the way it worked was that Toby's toys and beloved possessions naturally progressed to the downstairs playroom and Reuben claimed the bedroom as his play area throughout the day and holidays. They both needed somewhere separate to retreat to for quiet times. You can also achieve this with room dividers or anything that clearly demarcates an area of personal space.

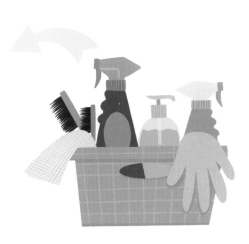

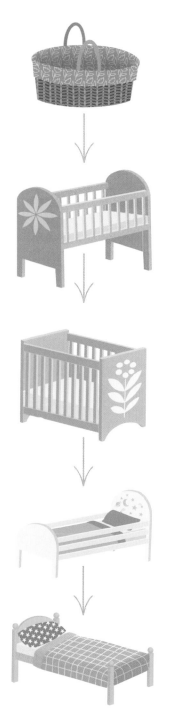

Decorating children's spaces

One of the things I learnt fairly quickly with my kids is that decorating their rooms can cost a fortune. You think you're just going to 'give it a little spruce up' and 'tweak a few things' and, before you know it, you've spent a fortune and are wondering how the hell it happened. You didn't spend this much on your own bedroom and your child doesn't even like bedtime.

It's not even something that you just do once in a blue moon either, is it? We do the nursery, then we spruce it up a bit for a toddler bedroom, then a child's bedroom and a tween bedroom and a teen bedroom and again... and again. It just keeps going, especially when we fall into the trap of decorating our child's bedroom to suit their current favourite characters.

However, decorating your child's bedroom doesn't have to be an expensive feat and, in fact, can be simple and last far longer than a mere couple of years.

According to a survey by Next Home in 2019, parents spend an average of £5,300 on a nursery and a further £4,500 before the child is aged 10. That's just shy of £10,000. On One Room.

How to create a nursery or bedroom that grows with your child

When we decorated Edith's bedroom, I accepted that I wouldn't be redecorating it any time soon as we were saving money to renovate and extend the ground floor. As I write this book, she is now five and a half and we haven't redecorated once since she was born, which is more than I can say for her brothers' rooms. There are few rooms in the house that we have spent so little on and that fit their 'owner' so well. It is one of the best rooms in the house (when it's clean and tidy, which of course it never is because, children). Here are my decoration tips.

THINK LONG TERM

During my time at Mothercare, when new parents were buying the first post-Moses basket cot bed for their baby, one of the things I would hear most often was 'but it looks too big, we'll get the smaller one'. Now, I grant you, a cot bed looks HUGE for a teeny tiny baby that you can still bundle up in your arms, but my god that cot bed will pay itself off in no time. A cot bed, in case you haven't heard the term, is a bed that converts from a cot to a small toddler bed without sides. They are usually a bit more expensive than cots, but cheaper than buying a cot and mattress, and then a toddler bed and mattress in two years' time because you don't think your little one should have a full single bed yet. One cot bed will last you until your child is around five years old, depending on their height, at which point you would switch to the next step.

Think long-term when buying furniture for your children and you won't regret it. FYI, long-term doesn't have to equate to expensive either. A lot of our furniture has come from Ikea or from the less-expensive baby retailers and it has lasted really well. The same is true for wardrobes and drawers. There are actually a lot of good options for changing tables that convert to a chest of drawers, or even a nice chest of drawers that you can then add a ridged side changing mat to. Regardless of whether you have a proper changing table with sides or a chest of drawers with a mat, you should never leave a baby or toddler alone on it. So, ask yourself why you're buying one instead of a normal long-lasting chest of drawers.

For that first bed, ask yourself if you want to keep changing it, and if the honest answer is that you don't mind and you have the budget, then cool. Go ahead and buy the bright pink princess fairy tale bed or the awesome car-shaped bed –whatever tickles your pickle. If you don't, think about a plain frame that they won't want to change for at least 5-8 years. Reuben and Toby both have Ikea loft beds, and I can't see them changing them until they are in their mid-teens at least, at which point they will probably want a double bed and will have much more room because of fewer toys and less of a desire to sit on the floor and play.

Places like IKEA are amazing for space-saving furniture that doesn't cost the earth. Think beyond the 'child section' and look at their design ideas for small apartments too.

FROM BABY TO CHILD WITH COLOUR

With Edith's bedroom, we chose a really neutral colour scheme with a twist. We chose a warm white and then, using painting tape, I created a block feature in a really deep rose colour on one wall. It wasn't the usual colour you would use for a nursery, not a standard 'baby colour' but it was one that would grow with her. Using inexpensive art prints from places like Etsy (worth its weight in gold and a great way to support small independent artists) I made the room feel suited to a baby or toddler and, keeping the same frames, we eventually swapped the artwork and we will do that again as she grows for minimal cost.

The same wasn't true for Reuben's nursery. We were new parents and we used a 'decor theme' from Mothercare that I loved, but that wore out quickly. We had the curtains, the bedding and the wall runner and it meant a full re-do was needed when it was time to redecorate and upgrade to a 'big boy room'. Ultimately, it cost more, ate up more time and we learnt our lesson.

Reuben and Toby now both have rooms, like Edith's, which are totally adaptable. Reuben's room has three horizontal coloured stripes on a feature wall and Toby has all white paint decorated with wall stickers (also worth their weight in gold for adding a punch of colour but being extremely adaptable).

BRILLIANT BEDDING

Bedding and cushions are another fabulous way to lift a room. You can find wonderfully colourful bedding, character bedding and all manner of awesome cushions that will give the room a different vibe instantly. High-street stores offer a range of great (and affordable) bedding – John Lewis surprised us with children's bedding that was really stylish and only a little more than the supermarket equivalent.

WALL STICKERS

are an affordable way to take a 'base room' painted in neutral colours and make it suitable for a range of ages and/or styles. Try looking on Etsy for small, independent sellers, they often have a huge variety of styles – be specific in your searches.

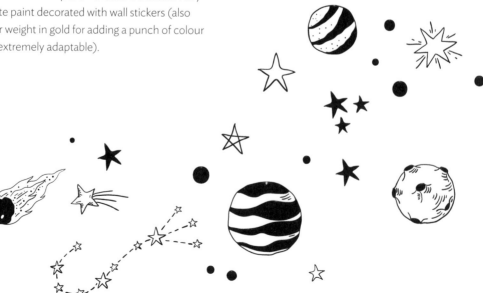

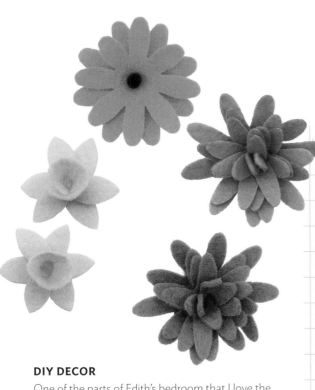

DIY DECOR

One of the parts of Edith's bedroom that I love the most are her curtains. At the time, we simply didn't have the budget to buy fancy curtains or blinds, so we improvised. We bought some curtains from Dunelm at a reduced price and then, using faux flowers from Hobbycraft and a glue gun, I created flower drop curtains for around £35. They suited her room as a baby/toddler and they still suit it now. She's due new furniture but the curtains and walls won't need to be touched. You can also use felt flowers, which you can buy from Etsy. I think I'll also keep the paper decorations that we saved some from her christening and hung on her walls as they look fab and she loves them – and I hardly spent a thing.

Invest in **BLACKOUT BLINDS** or curtains from the get-go. You will thank me later. The Gro Anywhere blind, while expensive, was one of the best things we bought for travelling and keeping the light out on sunny summer evenings.

Bedding woe-busters

Bed wetter? No problem. B-sensible fitted sheets by Sensible Sheets saved our sanity during night potty training. These sheets are soft and fit beautifully, while also being completely waterproof and eradicating the need for mattress protectors and those uncomfortable plastic sheets. You would never know they were different to 'normal' fitted sheets. We have them on all our beds, including mine and Adam's for those times the kids are sick or have an accident in our bed. https://sensiblesheets.co.uk

Does your child get tangled up in the duvet or kick it to the bottom of the cover? Marks & Spencer have created coverless, machine washable duvets. They only come in simple, neutral colours at the moment, but they will hopefully expand the range. Reuben really struggled with a duvet cover and every night we would find the duvet kicked to the bottom and he would wake up freezing, so this has totally revolutionised his sleeping.

HACK Got a duvet cover they prefer but they kick the duvet down? Stitch in some poppers from a craft or pound shop and stitch them into the corners of the duvet and duvet cover.

Playroom hacks

There is something to be said for a nice playroom. I flit between seeing the luxurious playrooms of Pinterest and Instagram and then the hideous reality of my own shit-show playroom, filled to the brim with kid's 'stuff' and their discarded clothes.

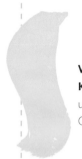

WIPEABLE BATHROOM OR KITCHEN PAINT We didn't use it and we regret it. Little Greene do a great matte range.

LAUNDRY BASKETS you no longer want are easily upcycled into toy boxes so don't get rid! **PICNIC HAMPERS** are great too if you don't have animals or very young children. Simply pop your toys in and sit back with a tidier room!

My kids are forever bring toy boxes from one place to another, so why not buy some **HEAVY DUTY WHEELS** from eBay and attach them to larger toy boxes to make them easier to move about for those times when the playroom simply won't do!

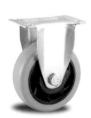

SIMPLE BLOCK FURNITURE (I'm a huge fan of Ikea's Kallax shelving unit) is perfect for toy storage. You can customise it with drawers from Etsy or eBay. The plastic drawers are stronger and longer lasting. Avoid wicker if you have pets or younger children as it can be a splinter hazard.

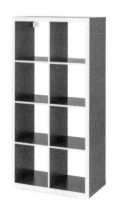

TOY BOXES If you're using 'lid' style toy boxes, then try getting some sticky-back foam strips for underneath the rim of the toy box lid. Not only will this stop that almighty bang that makes you wet yourself every time your kiddo drops the lid down, but it will also stop those horrible trapped-finger moments. We used to have a really deep chest that was once a bedroom chest and, when Toby was little, Reuben dropped the lid on him by accident. His poor little fingers were completely blue!

TENTS make amazing reading nooks, and they can be an investment piece in a playroom. When we were struggling to get Edith to do her work during the pandemic, she would sit in her tent and it helped her feel calmer. It became a permanent feature. If you don't want to buy a tent, create your own reading nook. There are so many different ideas for how to do this on Pinterest, ranging from the incredibly simple to the really extravagant – you can even use furniture and drapes.

LABEL MAKERS are a great way to help the kids remember where certain toys go. I bought one very cheaply from Amazon, and it has helped the older children to keep their rooms in some order, meaning I have less 'Mummmmm, where's my *insert obviously right in front of them or never-to-be-found-again item*?' Of course it doesn't stop them asking altogether, that would take a miracle, but it helps me say 'have you checked the XYZ drawer?'.

MUM HACK If you are looking for a large comfy floor cushion to fit into a tent or reading nook, I strongly recommend looking at... dog beds! Yes, I know it sounds ludicrous to suggest buying a dog bed for your child, but they are often a LOT cheaper than the Instagrammable 'floor cushion' and exactly the same thing. Save yourself some money, buy a neutral-coloured dog bed, and thank me later.

For little children, line the playroom floor with **FOAM PLAYMATS**. You can easily buy them online or in most shops in a range of colours and styles to suit your heart's desire. Simply cover the floor and cut them to fit flush. It's a great way to make a wipeable, safe surface for your young children to play on.

Create your own **CHALKBOARD.** When the boys were tiny, we dedicated a small portion of our living room as a play area with all their toys in. We created a 'chalkboard' by stripping the wallpaper off a corner of wall, then painted the wall with chalkboard paint. They loved it. If you don't fancy painting your walls, a piece of wood (perhaps the old backing of a frame) would be perfect. Attach to the wall and away you go.

You're never too young to appreciate a bit of artwork! Don't shy away from **ART ON THE WALLS**. You can find some wonderful, fun art prints from small sellers at places like Etsy. From the inspiring girl power prints to the fun animal prints, let the walls talk!

Their style, your home

When Reuben was little and went into his first bed, I remember having a conversation with my husband about what to buy him. Adam wanted to get him some character bedding that he loved and paint his wall with a fancy mural or use posters and I just hated the idea – it's just not my style. I wanted to create a room that I would love and he would love too.

The thing I would say about decorating a child's space is that it's still your home, your money and ultimately your say. If you aren't keen on something, don't buy it just because your child will love it – that is what their toys are for. Look outside of the box: a lot of shops that cater to children's everything – toys, clothes and interior – are very limited in what they offer. Don't stick to exclusively high street or only the children's ranges either.

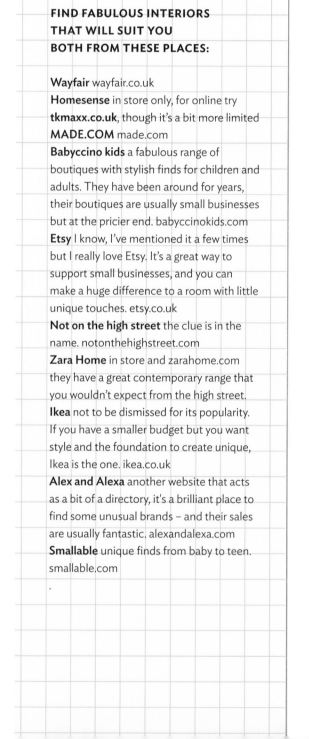

FIND FABULOUS INTERIORS THAT WILL SUIT YOU BOTH FROM THESE PLACES:

Wayfair wayfair.co.uk

Homesense in store only, for online try **tkmaxx.co.uk**, though it's a bit more limited

MADE.COM made.com

Babyccino kids a fabulous range of boutiques with stylish finds for children and adults. They have been around for years, their boutiques are usually small businesses but at the pricier end. babyccinokids.com

Etsy I know, I've mentioned it a few times but I really love Etsy. It's a great way to support small businesses, and you can make a huge difference to a room with little unique touches. etsy.co.uk

Not on the high street the clue is in the name. notonthehighstreet.com

Zara Home in store and zarahome.com they have a great contemporary range that you wouldn't expect from the high street.

Ikea not to be dismissed for its popularity. If you have a smaller budget but you want style and the foundation to create unique, Ikea is the one. ikea.co.uk

Alex and Alexa another website that acts as a bit of a directory, it's a brilliant place to find some unusual brands – and their sales are usually fantastic. alexandalexa.com

Smallable unique finds from baby to teen. smallable.com

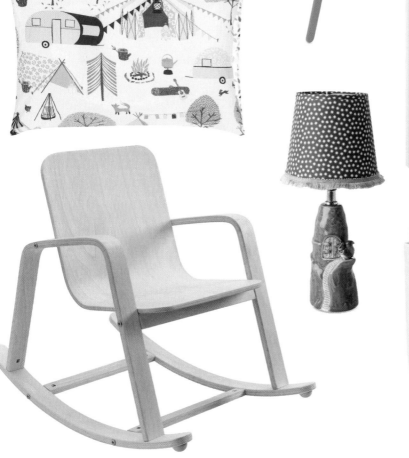
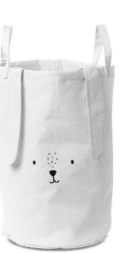

Tidy home, tidy mind (sort of)

True to a degree, I'll grant you, but not for me the 'be all and end all'. Sometimes, that tidy home is just beyond us and, after an long day of work or whatever we have been doing, the last thing the majority of us want to do is cleaning. Frankly, it often falls into the 'weekend task' category for us and, when we do get to the point where we have the time to actually crack on, it's the last thing we want to do. Weekends are for family time and relaxing, not for scrubbing out the shower or washing all the kitchen cupboards. Then, unfortunately, comes the frustration because I hate mess and clutter, and my husband is the same. I let my annoyance build and then BOOM, there is a falling out over who should have done what and when, despite it never being mentioned. Neither of us possess psychic abilities to communicate how much we wanted the other to 'Hinch' the house... or at least scrub the fecking toilet.

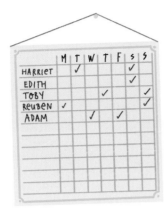

I'll lay it out for you, I always thought I HATED cleaning with a passion. I thought my husband would be the one who (reluctantly) handled those household chores while I cracked on with the cooking, the putting IN of laundry (never putting it away though because that is truly a task I hate *shudders*) and the life admin that comes with being an adult. In reality, I don't actually hate cleaning as much as I thought I did. I hate the thought of cleaning far more than the reality. I look around my house, see my kids undoing the cleaning and tidying I've done or the pets shedding fur and it just feels completely insurmountable. Yet, with the rise of cleaning influencers making it look so *easy*, I feel pressured to get something done half of the time and Marie Kondo-ing my kids is not an option.

With that in mind, I worked out a way to hack my cleaning and this means that I really don't spend as much time on it as you might think. I also cut back on spending a fortune and introducing lots of chemicals into the house. Please don't get me wrong, I'm a big chemical fan when it's necessary and *actually* works, but sometimes, the natural way is just... the better way.

How to prioritise cleaning your home

The first thing you should know about cleaning is that it's a constant juggle. However, it doesn't actually have to be a real pain in the arse and 90 per cent of the time you're doing it a lot more than you think. It also takes a lot less time if you're keeping on top of it.

'Is it actually messy?' is the first thing you need to be asking yourself. Does this space really need cleaning? I always prioritise the areas where I'm going to be cooking or serving food, so my kitchen and dining space, followed by bathrooms, because no one wants to go there. We spend a lot of time in the living room so that usually comes next, with beds and bedrooms afterwards (no one sees them if they come over) and finally, the hallway spaces.

Before cleaning influencers really became a 'thing' I was a big fan of Gemma from The Organised Mum who created a method known as TOMM. Using a simple schedule, this helps you to prioritise your cleaning and reduce it down to 30 minutes a day. It's a really good way to maintain some balance but have a reasonably clean and tidy home.

Hack your kitchen

TRYING TO GET BURNS OFF THE BOTTOM OF A HIDEOUSLY BURNT PAN? There is nothing worse than scrubbing away or putting the pan through a dishwasher cycle only to find it still there at the end. Try soaking the pan in Coca Cola for a minimum of four hours, preferably overnight, then wash as normal.

MESH BAGS are an ideal way to keep all the little bits and bobs, like baby spoons or children's plastic toys (Lego!) together in your dishwasher. Did I also mention that your dishwasher is an amazing place to wash your kid's grotty bath toys? It is.

WOODEN CHOPPING BOARDS have become super popular once again, but the one thing that they are is difficult to clean as they absorb the smells of whatever you use – and no one wants their food chopped on something with the lingering flavour of toxic chemicals do they? Grab yourself a lemon wedge covered in salt, rub around the chopping board and then wipe clean with warm water.

STINKY BIN Let's face it, bins stink and so investing in a good bin with a lid is always going to help. However, also try cleaning your bin by sprinkling with baking powder and then rubbing down with half a lemon before rinsing in water. Or, if you prefer, use Method Anti-bac All Purpose Cleaner in Orange Yuzu or Sunny Citrus as citrus smells help to banish other scents. Finally, when you put a new bin liner in, add a few drops of essential oil to a piece of kitchen paper. Drop this into the bottom of the bin and be amazed at the lack of smell!

POLISH STAINLESS STEEL WITH... FLOUR Yes, flour. I know, it's weird but it works. Wash and dry your stainless steel sink or your taps as usual, then sprinkle with a small amount of flour and buff with a dry cloth. It will leave everything sparkling clean.

FRIDGE SMELLS I have to confess I frequently have a stinky fridge because I love me some stinky cheeses. My fave way to banish fridge smells is to drop vanilla essence onto some cotton wool and place it in a dish in your fridge together with some orange or lemon peel. Does it always banish the worst smells? No, but it will give your fridge a lovely smell 98 per cent of the time. **While we're talking fridges, a damp natural sponge placed in your veg drawer keeps veggies and fruit crisp.**

MY FAVOURITE FLOOR CLEANING SOLUTION is Zoflora. It smells amazing and comes in so many scents. It's also really inexpensive and has a million and one uses. It cleans my house and sets a long-lasting smell which helps to create a real vibe – especially at Christmas time when I order cinnamon, winter spice and mulled wine scents. It costs less than candles and lasts almost as long.

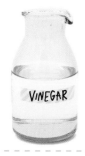

If you're looking for a **NATURAL AND EVEN CHEAPER WAY TO CLEAN YOUR KITCHEN FLOORS,** mix 2 cups (500ml) of white distilled vinegar with 6 cups (1.5l) of warm water – an anti-bac, suitable for counters and floors.

LIMESCALE IN THE KETTLE CAN BE PARTIALLY SOLVED WITH A PEBBLE We bought a lovely glass kettle for our new kitchen and the limescale build up ruined it, literally within a day of having it. We popped a pebble inside so we don't have to fill it with descaler every other day. Or a better piece of advice is to avoid a glass kettle...

WOODEN FLOORS AND TILES? Ditch the mop and buy a Bissell CrossWave 3-in-1 Multicleaner. It's pricey, but it acts as a vacuum, mop and floor drier all in one, plus it's suitable for both wood and tiles, unlike the mop. Spend that extra and you won't regret it.

SOAK YOUR DISH CLOTHS (always try to get microfibre) in the sink overnight in a capful of Zoflora and water. I was sceptical when this was recommended by popular cleaning guru 'Mrs Hinch' but it works and makes the kitchen smell wonderful.

CLEANING YOUR OVEN Oven Pride is a longterm favourite of mine, but it's something that I always mean to do, and then I trot off to bed, forgetting to soak it overnight as you need to. Obviously cleaning up new spills as soon as they occur is ideal, but does anyone really do that when their kids are barking 'when's dinner ready?!' No, of course not. You can use dishwasher powder to clean your oven if those pesky spills dry. Simply wet the spills, cover in dishwasher powder and cover in wet kitchen paper – it really does work!

TOOTHBRUSHES ARE THE UNSUNG CLEANING TOOL when it comes to tiles and cleaning the grout between them. The Pink Stuff is also excellent for cleaning grout.

WATER STAINS ON THE HOB Nothing is quite as annoying as water stains on a hob and I can never ever get them out with normal cleaning solutions – even Cif and The Pink Stuff fails me. However, bicarbonate of soda, mixed into a toothpaste-like consistency with a little water and left on the water stain for a minimum of 15 minutes, then wiped off with a cloth, does the trick. You might have to scrub the bicarb into the stain a bit if it is a really old one, but it will lift it eventually.

Hack your bathroom

THROW OUT THE TOILET BRUSH This is one of the most common bathroom and downstairs WC items, but it is possibly the most unhygienic. My mother-in-law swears by not having one and I agree – when you think about it, they are never actually clean. Get yourself a good pair of marigolds and a scrubbing sponge that can either be washed in the machine or binned.

MILDEW ON THE SHOWER CURTAIN?
A great way to stop this from building up is giving it a wash every week and allowing it to dry. However, if you're still finding it building up and you don't want to buy a new one, add ½ cup (90g) of bicarbonate of soda to your washing, then wash at 30°C. Before your rinse cycle, add ½ cup (125ml) of vinegar.

TO HELP MAKE YOUR BATHROOM SMELL NICE
add some essential oil to the cardboard inside your toilet roll. You only need a few drops so it doesn't sink through the paper and come into contact with the skin. However, these few drops will release a little more scent with every twist of the roll.

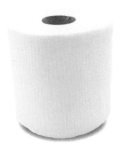

SCRUB A DUB TUB
Clean your bathtub with half a grapefruit heavily coated in salt. It will remove both greasy residue and water marks. Rinse with warm water.

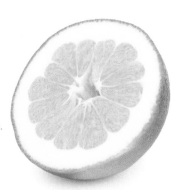

BLOCKED DRAINS ARE AN ABSOLUTE NIGHTMARE Start by using a plunger to see if you can 'dislodge' anything. You can also try using boiling water to see if whatever you have blocking your drain is fat-based, though this is usually for a kitchen drain. Finally, baking powder and vinegar can sometimes help. Use ⅓ (110g) cup of baking powder, followed by ½ cup (125ml) of vinegar and *quickly* put the plug in the sink. The baking powder and vinegar create that 'volcano' explosion you often see used in school projects and can sometimes dissolve blockages. Wait 30 minutes and then pour hot water down the sink. Mr Muscle Max Gel Unblocker is a product that can tackle blockages too.

CLEANING SHOWER GLASS Our shower doors are an absolute nightmare – the blunt truth is that we don't have the time or inclination to wipe them down after every use, though to be honest we would make our lives so much easier if we did. However, a steam cleaner (the Karcher Handheld WV10 Steam Cleaner) is brilliant for making light work of wiping down those water-marked shower doors and windows.

LIMESCALE ON THE SHOWER? Not a problem – wrap kitchen paper (or cloths) around your shower and soak in distilled white vinegar. Leave for an hour and rinse. Repeat if necessary.

GROSS TOILET? Ours is horrendous with three males, two of whom can't seem to grasp the concept of the sit down if it's the 'pee everywhere' wee. It needs a regular clean and by that I mean daily. Harpic is a brilliant toilet cleaner, but to remove brown stains, use a litre of vinegar, leave for three hours or overnight, scrub with a scrubbing sponge and flush the toilet. Repeat if needed.

USE A SCREWDRIVER OR DINNER KNIFE WRAPPED IN A WIPE OR CLOTH to get between the body of your toilet and tank, and underneath the seat. Don't flush wipes as they contribute to blocked drains.

WALL MEDICINE CABINETS are a great way to use up some wall space and keep your bathroom nice and tidy looking. If you have the room, a tower shelving unit is ideal for popping baskets on to store all of your bathroom products. Add a little hook to the side to hang your jewellery while you have a bath or shower.

ADD A PING PONG BALL TO YOUR TOILET to help little boys concentrate on where to pee. This will hopefully cut back on the amount of urine you have to clean up on your floors...

CLEANING BATHROOM MIRRORS IS REALLY EASY WITH VINEGAR!
Just a touch of vinegar topped up with water in a spray bottle will bring up a real sparkle. You can also try some glass cleaner solution and, if you want to stop them from steaming up, use some shaving foam to polish after cleaning.

SWEET-SMELLING SINK Wash out your sink as you would normally, then dry. Put some of your favourite-smelling Zoflora onto a dry cloth or piece of kitchen paper and wipe around your dry sink. This works especially well on stone sink but will work on anything and leaves a lovely smell in your bathroom.

Hack your living room

WINNING WINDOWS If you're looking for a natural window cleaner, then use a 50/50 solution of vinegar and warm water. However, avoid cleaning on sunny days as the solution dries too quickly and leaves streaks behind. Polish up with a paper coffee filter or lint-free cloth to avoid little bits of fabric being left on the windows.

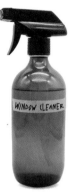

PET BED Pet beds are something that I have a love/hate relationship with – they keep the pets off my sofas but they can really stink after a time, especially if you have one that isn't machine washable. Spray your pet bed with a natural deodoriser of baking powder, essential oil and water. Be careful with essential oils though – lavender can be toxic to cats so check before you use it. Finally, if you're unlucky enough to find your pet picks up fleas, you will need to spray their bedding with a good de-fleaing spray from the vets. You can wrap a hot water bottle wrapped in double-sided sticky tape and drag it across the bed. The fleas will leap into the air to avoid the heat and attach themselves to the tape.

SOFA CARE Grab yourself a sofa stain kit when you buy a sofa. Most places that sell sofas will offer you one, but request one if not.

Daily sofa care: Flip cushions and give them a daily plumping by patting them on both sides and dropping on a clean floor.
Weekly sofa care: Wipe your sofa with a dry or damp cloth, depending on the fabric, and follow it up with a brush with a clothes brush. We have a velvet sofa and this helps to keep its colour and lift the crushed fibres. Use up leftover fabric softener to create a homemade freshener. Simply place that small, leftover amount in a spray bottle and top up with water, then spritz sparingly onto your sofa. However, be careful about new jeans on light fabric sofas – the dye may transfer.

BOBBLES/FABRIC PILLS on woollen sofas are easily sorted with a fabric shaver, but if you don't have one, a pair of clippers used with care are excellent alternatives.

DUSTING No duster, no problem. A pair of old opaque tights can be repurposed to collect dust. They create a static and pick up dust better than most fibre cloths.

CANDLES create a wonderful ambience and are at the top of my list of 'me treats'. For unbelievable scent, try Sand + Fog or thisworks candles. Also, if you pop your candle in a freezer for 24 hours before you burn it, it will last almost double the time!

SQUEAKY DOORS I have the best intentions to turn our shed into a well-stocked and organised DIY shrine, but in reality it resembles Monica's closet rather than anything useful. So, my husband came up with a way to fix the squeaky doors in our house without the likes of WD40 (which is great, if you have it). If you are stuck with squeaky hinges, for a quick fix, grab a bottle of hairspray and spray the hinge while moving it back and forth. Leave for a few minutes and check – the squeak should be gone!

Add a drop of your favourite essential oil to a dry cloth and wipe around your cold (switched off) **LIGHT BULBS**, then leave to dry. When you switch on the lights, your living room will smell wonderful.

TO DUST YOUR TV WITHOUT DAMAGING THE SCREEN use a TV screen cleaner – or if you don't have one, use a paper coffee filter. It does the same job, and even picks up the fibre specks that screen cleaners leave behind.

KEEP YOUR TV REMOTE CONTROL CLEAN with a small dollop of hand sanitiser on a kitchen towel. Remove the batteries and gently wipe all over.

RUG LIFE When we first did up the house, one of the things that I searched high and low for was a rug to tie the living room together. We don't have a beautiful, plush carpet because we thought it better to be safe than sorry with young children and pets, but I wanted a rug to give something of the same effect. I fell in love with a beautiful cream one (oh how foolish can I be?), and so over the years I've had to learn various ways to deal with its many trials and tribulations.

Washing – if suitable, pop it straight in the washing machine but, if not, hang the rug across a washing line and soak with a hosepipe, then use washing-up liquid on any stains and allow to dry in the sunshine. However, be warned, if it's an expensive rug or something very delicate, leave it to the pros.

Spot cleaning – for any stains that you see happen (like a spillage or a dropped piece of food) clean immediately with a multi-purpose cleaner, if you have one. If not, place a small amount of vinegar on a soft cloth and dab, never rub.

Bobbles/fabric pills – get yourself a fabric shaver; it will become worth its weight in gold.

Weekly refresh – spruce up your rug with a cleaner, like 1001 Carpet Fresh, for minimal fuss and no vacuuming. Or, if you prefer a natural alternative, sprinkle a little bicarbonate of soda and a few drops of essential oil over your rug, leave to sit for 15 minutes, and then vacuum up.

Hack your
bedrooms

KEEP BEDDING IN A PILLOWCASE ONCE IT'S BEEN FOLDED then you will never lose the matching pillowcases for your duvet sets!

FLIP (or rotate) **YOUR MATTRESS** once a month in order to keep the springs intact. Ideally, a mattress needs replacing every 7-10 years.

Save space in your wardrobe by **VACUUM PACKING CLOTHES** by 'season'. Bulky jumpers can be vacuum packed and put away in the wardrobe or under the bed during summer. I buy packs of three different sized vacuum bags from Amazon and stuff them full of my jumpers then attach the nozzle of my vacuum cleaner (just without any head on the tube) to the fitting in the bag and switch it on!

SILK PILLOWS sound like an unnecessary luxury but they actually have a purpose beyond feeling decadent. The natural properties of silk can help to limit the friction caused to your hair when you are sleeping, so it's ideal for preventing split ends and helping to reduce frizz. On top of this, it's great for helping to keep your skin healthy.

To clean any **SMELLS ON YOUR MATTRESS** without chemicals, pop some vodka in a spray bottle and add a few drops of essential oil. Spray lightly across the offending area and leave to air dry. It won't remove stains but it should help with busting the smell if your child had an accident or an illness.

Use a pair of braces to **KEEP FITTED SHEETS IN PLACE.** You can buy fitted sheet clips, but a pair of braces will work just as well. To attach the braces, lift your mattress to show the underside of your fitted sheet then clip one side to the horizontal side of your bed and one to the vertical side, going across your corner to hold in place. Simple!

Tie a couple of **TENNIS BALLS** into an old sock and throw this into the dryer along with your bedsheets. This will help them to dry evenly – no more half-dry sheets!

PILLOW SPRAY can be really useful for helping promote sleep. You can buy sprays or diffuser oils and I love NEOM's Perfect Night essential oil mix. Alternatively, place a few drops of lavender essential oil on a tissue and tuck it into your pillowcase. This is better than dropping the oil directly onto bed linen as it can stain.

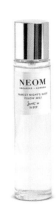

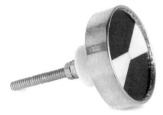

Transform furniture with ease by simply changing the **HANDLES.** You can find beautiful handles on places like Etsy and eBay and it totally uplifts a basic, inexpensive chest of drawers.

LIGHT plays a huge part in our sleep patterns! Blackout curtains are great for helping to block out external light, but in the bedroom your lighting is equally important. Try a light diffusing pendant light shade for your ceiling lights, and warm, yellow toned light bulbs for your bedside lamps.

Bed linen ideally needs washing once a week, and **THERE IS NOTHING LIKE CLIMBING INTO FRESH BED SHEETS!** To add a gorgeous long-lasting scent, throw some Lenor Unstoppables or other scent boosters into your wash, and then place a scented dryer sheet in between your folded sheets. To make your own, take a muslin square and spray lightly with your favourite perfume, then leave to dry and fold.

Instead of a traditional alarm clock, try out a gradual wake up **SUNRISE LAMP**. The light will gradually come on at a time of your choosing and wake you up in a much more calming way. Sleep cycle app is also great for gradually waking you up and tracking your sleep patterns to help you learn how to get the best night's sleep you can.

FAKE TAN STAINS They are a nightmare aren't they? There are only so many times that the stains will come out of light bedding. I recommend putting your tan on first thing in the morning and, if you fake tan in the evening, wash your sheets the following day, even if there is no stain. You can use a stain remover, like Vanish Gold, or add ½ cup (125ml) bleach to a bucket of hot water, and then presoak for 30-60 minutes before washing on the highest setting your sheets will take.

Laundry life

No one, and I mean *no one* makes a mess of clothes like a child does and, really, my kids take the biscuit. If it's not messy eating, it's messy play and I'm partly to blame as I wholeheartedly encourage it. It's one of those things that you can do as a kid and that, sadly, isn't such a part of adult life, and so stains are just something I've accepted I have to deal with...

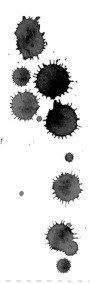

BLOOD Scraped knees or nose bleeds, whatever the blood stain, the easiest way to get rid of it is to soak the offending item for an hour in ¼ cup (75g) of salt and enough hot water to cover the garment completely. For older blood stains, try using a stain remover and gently rubbing with a toothbrush, or use a meat tenderizer paste (the enzymes break down the blood) mixed with a little water. Leave to dry and brush off before washing as normal.

YELLOW ARMPIT STAINS The bane of the white shirt, especially for tweens/teens who are hormonal and have just started using deodorant, but they can also happen to anyone. I use a liquid peroxide soak (obviously white garments only) and then wash on the hottest setting and this sometimes shifts these pesky stains.

GRASS STAINS Probably the most common (and annoying) stain in our house. Make a solution of two parts hot water to one part distilled white vinegar and soak the stain for 15 minutes. Dab the stain gently and then wash using an enzyme-based laundry detergent. **MUM TIP:** These types of laundry detergents work better on a low temperature setting. In the past, I put my heavily stained items in a high temperature wash – big mistake.

LET'S GET MUDDY (OR NOT) Mud is usually one that just comes right out, but sometimes it can be a nightmare to get out of Toby's cricket whites or football gear. In my experience, this is one for the detergents. I like to use a good enzyme-based liquid detergent and place it neat onto the stain, then soak for an hour. If you want to try something else, mix bicarbonate of soda with a little water to create a paste and then apply this to the offending area. Allow to soak before washing as normal.

POSTER PAINT, AKA THE DEVIL I will level with you, this is tougher to deal with than strapping an unwilling toddler into a car seat. Reuben's preschool clothes were relentlessly stained with poster paint and while I used to have 'painting clothes' that were a mismatch of partially outgrown and stained clothes, poster paint is hell to remove. The only thing I've ever found that *mostly* removes the stain is a bar of hand soap and COLD water.

CLEANING YOUR WASHING MACHINE

is a priority. It's no use trying to clean clothes with something dirty is it? Wipe down your doors and inside using vinegar on a microfibre cloth, fill the clean and empty detergent compartment with vinegar and run on a hot setting. If you think your machine could use a boost, use 1/3 cup (60g) of bicarbonate of soda in the drum of your washing machine and run the machine on the hottest setting one more time. Never, ever use disinfectants in your machine that aren't approved as they could cause serious damage!

TOMATO STAINS Nothing fills me with quite as much joy as seeing my beloved children slurp down the Spag Bol I have made for them, but it is the messiest darn food I have ever known, and I challenge anyone to try and convince a nine year old that he should wear a bib to eat. Anyway, Fairy Liquid (or any other washing-up soap) is your friend! Wet the stain, rub in some soap and then, as you're rubbing, rinse under cold water. Once you have removed as much stain as possible, wash as normal and repeat the process if needed.

INK BLOTCHES I've lost count of the amount of times the kids have accidentally inked themselves. Acetate-free hairspray can help – spray the area, leave for 10 minutes and rinse. For white school shirts, Place 1 teaspoon of salt on to half a lemon and scrub into the white shirt then soak the lot (lemon, salt and shirt) in enough hot water to cover for 5–10 minutes before washing.

Spray a muslin cloth with your favourite perfume or air freshener and place in your laundry basket to avoid those **MUSTY CLOTHES SMELLS.** Especially useful if you have sport-loving people in the house. Alternatively, use one of those drawer liners that is designed to make your cupboards and drawers smell nice.

FOUNDATION AND MAKE UP

STAINS I have this gorgeous white dress and, for the life of me, I can't help but get foundation stains around the neck. It's a fairly high-neck dress and it became cooked in there and was driving me bonkers. However, I found a hack online for removing it and I was really sceptical at first, but it works. Apply neat shaving foam (any brand, just make sure it's foam) and leave it for a few minutes. Rinse and repeat if necessary. Wash the item as normal and voila!

BABY POO Yup, the one that curses us all. You think you're just going about your day and BOOM – poonami. These little buggers are even more of a pain if you are a cloth nappy user. Firstly, you need to make sure the area is *actual poo* free. Then rinse and spray with a solution of 1/4 cup (60 ml) lemon juice to 1 cup (250 ml) water. Scrub the area with a toothbrush or something with bristles and then let it sit for 15 minutes. Wash as you normally would and dry in direct sunlight.

Let's talk chores

When I first became a mum, I never really thought of chores as something that was a controversial or debatable topic. Your kids live in the house, they will one day have to live alone – be that at uni or when they move out – and it's sensible to teach them how to run a house, right?

Well, apparently it isn't that simple. There are endless opinions about chores (surprise surprise, isn't that the case with everything in parenthood?), from which chores are bad for kids to which are good for kids, and when they should start doing them. I think, as with all things parenting, there is one thing to remember: **do what works for you**.

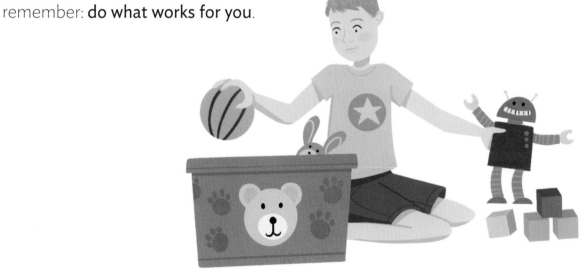

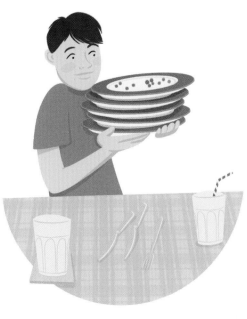

Do what works for you

In every family set up there will be a different way of doing things, and what Karen down the road thinks you should do is irrelevant, as is what your parents tell you that you had to do as a child. The task is to work out what works FOR YOU and run with it. It will take a bit of fiddling about, but once you find something that you're happy with, stick with it and add to it gradually. I think it's really important to note that 'chore' doesn't necessarily mean what it used to. When I was a child, a chore was something like hoovering or collecting all the laundry and loading the washing machine. It was about a child owning a bit of responsibility and helping with simple tasks. Nowadays I think we have a much broader idea of chores than a child simply doing small things like keeping their spaces tidy and picking up toys.

In our house, from an early age, our children have helped out with simple things like clearing the table after a meal and tidying toys and then, as they have gotten a little older, we've encouraged them to help us with more and more. We've also encouraged their natural preferences. Edith, for example, loves to load the dishwasher and switch it on and she also enjoys sorting the laundry into the right colours and putting on a load. Reuben, on the other hand, prefers preparing food and will happily go into the kitchen and make himself basic meals or snacks if he is hungry. I'm under absolutely no illusion that this will last beyond the age of 13 and beyond then they will all probably resent being asked to do anything that isn't entirely self-serving, BUT at the moment, it's a great foundation to have.

Incentives + chores

Do you expect children to do chores for a reward, or just because they are a part of the family and it's important that everyone has a role to play? Well, I think that's another one for the ol 'do what works for you' line. There are so many ways to reward children for doing simple tasks and, if you want a financial incentive, try using services like Go Henry, where they have their own bank card and you give them a certain amount of pocket money every week. The amount depends on whether they complete all the tasks you set for them on the app and, if you want to give them something extra, you can transfer across more money with a few clicks. If you want to avoid money incentives, why not set up a visual board where they can work towards earning a trip somewhere. Ultimately, it has to be up to you.

Home tasks that the kids can help with

AGES 4-6
Picking up toys
Watering plants
Helping to clear the table after meals
Making the bed
Putting laundry upstairs in their bedrooms
    (unlikely they will be able to put
    it away at 4)

AGES 7-10
Putting laundry away/folding laundry
Putting a load of laundry in the wash
Loading the dishwasher/washing dishes
Drying dishes and putting them away
Dusting
Washing skirting boards
Making easy snacks
Helping make dinner/peeling vegetables
Helping clean the car inside and out
Cleaning out small pet cages
Sweeping/hoovering and/or mopping
Bringing empty bins inside (depending
    on home location/roads, etc)

AGES 11+
Emptying indoor bins
Cleaning stairs
Feeding pets
Ironing clothes (supervised)
Mowing lawns (supervised)
Cooking meals
Helping with home repairs/DIY

WHILST WE'RE ON THE SUBJECT

make your own list

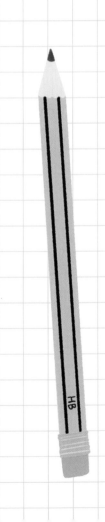

notes

TRAVEL

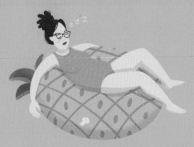

Travelling was never really a passion of mine until recently, and certainly after I had the kids. When I was in my late teens and early twenties, I had friends hopping all over the globe for 'years out', visiting Thailand, moving to Australia for a couple of years and living it up while they were young and seeing the world. I can honestly say, it never appealed to me. While my friends were dreaming of travels or off doing it, I was dreaming of decorating my own home, settling down with a partner to love, who would love me and a brood of at least five children. Yes, you read that right, at least five children – and then I had my three and realised that it's a bit harder than the image I conjured in my innocent 19-year-old noggin. However, I certainly didn't fancy the idea of travelling – working at carnivals or picking fruit to be able to afford the next hostel bed and never having the security of knowing where I was going to be next week or even the month after, just a rough plan and a backpack. I always felt a bit confused by it all and, to be honest, it was my idea of hell.

Then I hit thirty and the travel bug hit me with a vengeance.

Don't get me wrong, I still think that the young-adult version of backpacking or travelling from one spot to the next without much of a plan or financial security sounds like hell. I'm a meticulous planner and, while I've become really good at being more adventurous and spontaneous – the thought of hopping in the car and just driving somewhere doesn't fill me with the panic it used to – I now have the luxury of knowing that I have insurance, contingency plans and the ability to say 'sod it, let's go home' if something goes wrong. These are the securities that I simply couldn't afford as a young adult.

When you add children into the mix, people often become more anxious of travelling. They view it as a 'pre-kids' activity that, with kids, is just too much to cope with. I'm the reverse. Give me an airport, three small kids and all their luggage and I will be fine. Whether it is abroad or a staycation, it's something that I plan constantly. In fact, while still on holiday, I like to plan our next holiday. I'm the mum that says things like, 'Wouldn't it be amazing if we could tour Europe in one of those huge American caravans during the school six-week holiday?', while Adam scowls at me and my newfound wildness/total lack of practical thinking. He, by contrast, isn't that fussed – he enjoys it, but also loves being at home and simply relaxing.

However, I hope this section inspires you to travel more with your children. **As we get older, we don't look back on material things, we remember moments and time spent together.**

Travelling
with kids

Regardless of where you are going, it's often the getting there that stresses parents out the most. How will your kids cope with five hours in a car? Will they scream all the way to America on a plane? Will they be safe on board a ship?

Admittedly, travelling with children does sound daunting, but often it isn't as bad as you fear. I say 'often' as of course sometimes it **is** rubbish and there is nothing anyone can do. No matter how well prepared you are or how many blog posts you have read about making your child super-happy during a long-haul flight, sometimes it doesn't go to plan. However, having a plan definitely helps with a lot.

The first time we took Edith on a long-haul flight, she was 18 months old and I spent the majority of the time walking and breastfeeding her across the Atlantic. It was tiring but, overall, it wasn't too bad. I had planned ahead – yay me! The way back was a COMPLETELY different story – a nightmare. It was a night flight, the cabin crew weren't great and, unbeknownst to us, Edith had picked up hand, foot and mouth disease at our resort which only presented when we were an hour off the ground. Cue lots of panicking and staff trying to find a doctor to understand what the hell this random rash was, because she had been fine on the ground, just teething... My point? It won't always be smooth sailing but don't let it put you off.

Travelling by car

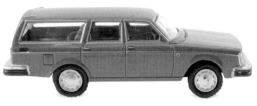

Travelling by car isn't discussed as much as travelling by plane but I'd say it can be a great way to go on holiday. We've had some really positive travels with the kids in the car, both up to North Yorkshire and down to Cornwall, and taking on a huge trip to the Vendée region of France.

THERE ARE A FEW REAL POSITIVES TO TRAVELLING TO YOUR HOLIDAY DESTINATION BY CAR, BE IT ABROAD OR AT HOME

You can fill your car FULL of snacks, blankets, clothes... pretty much anything.

You can stop as often as you like.

You don't have to be around other people, just you and your family unit, which means you can control what is on the radio, the temperature and whether or not you sing Vengaboys at the top of your lungs without being prosecuted for creating a disturbance.

You'll see things you absolutely wouldn't have seen with another method of travel. Driving across France was amazing because we drove all around the small islands near where we stayed, and discovered so many amazing little towns and villages that were beautiful and really only known by locals.

THERE ARE ALSO A FEW DRAWBACKS

It's slow. It can be reeeeally slow, depending on traffic.

No toilet – of course, you can stop, but the sudden 'I need a weeeeeeee!!!!' on the motorway will strike fear into any parent's heart. Keep an old plastic bottle in your car for boys to wee in. Girls tend to be better at holding it in (that's my experience).

It's a confined space so, if your kids are fighting, it's a pain, but at least you're not around other people...

It means one of you will need to be awake and alert enough to concentrate on driving, which is exhausting and often takes a bit of recovery.

Getting the best out of travelling with kids in the car:

Comfortable and age-appropriate car seats are a must. Get a trained car seat fitter to check your car seat or contact your local fire station and ask them if this is a service they offer – it frequently is.

Snacks, snacks and more snacks. Try to avoid lots and lots of sugar and sweets. Little and often is my motto, and don't forget drinks!

Plan frequent stops. When we travelled to Cornwall, we planned a route that allowed us lots of breaks, some overnight too. We stopped at Woburn Safari Park for a day out and spent the night at a Premier Inn, then carried on to Devon where we spent a few days at a campsite, and finally moved on to Cornwall for four days. When it was time to come back, we stopped about half way and spent the night at a hotel. It breaks it up when you're driving for over six hours. If you don't want to stop overnight, leave pre-5 am to make a good start and stop for breakfast between 8–9 am to avoid the worst of rush hour.

Entertainment is a must. We always make sure we have tablets with us, wherever we travel (don't forget chargers), as well as colouring books and magazines. Unfortunately, driving is the one method of travel where these are likely to make you feel really queasy! Audiobooks are amazing for long car journeys; they don't bring on sickness and even entertain the driver.

Pack a small bag of toys such as animal figures, cars or dolls. Break out a toy when they are bored!

Car seat travel trays. Perfect for children who want to do some colouring or need something to rest their tablet or book on. Readily available from Amazon, there are so many brands but I recommend LenBest as it has a place to store pens, toys and books/paper and a dry eraser top. WIN. Whatever you go for, be really careful to ensure it doesn't get attached around your child's car seat and potentially block their seat belt or buckle in the event of an accident or should you need to remove them from the seat quickly.

FREE GAMES FOR KIDS TO PLAY IN THE CAR
I-spy
Spot the car by colour – keep count of who spots each colour first to work out who wins
License plate game – pick a letter, find a license plate with it
Alphabet game – pick a topic and find a word that relates to that topic for every letter of the alphabet
Mini Cheddar – each player gets 1 point for spotting a Mini, 5 points for a yellow car, and 10 points for a yellow Mini

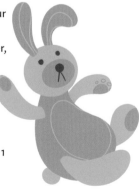

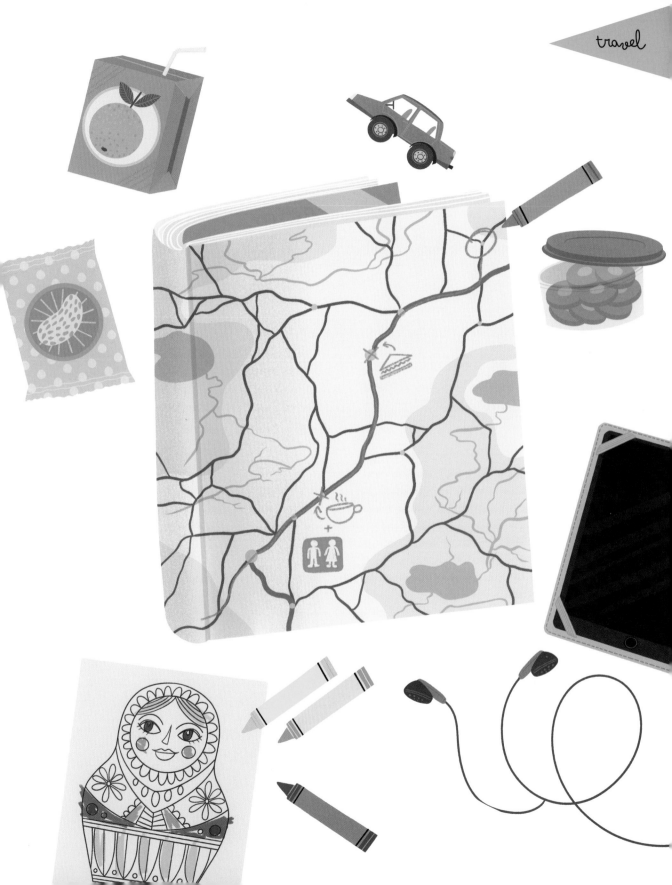

travel

Travelling by boat

It took me a while to convince Adam to travel by ferry with the kids and, despite being significantly safer than travelling by car, it's still his least favourite method of travel. His main reason, he admits, is his worry that they might fall overboard! This always makes me chuckle because it's just so unlikely, but we'll keep working on him (and about that cruise!).

The last time we travelled by ferry was from Hull to Rotterdam and onwards to Efteling in the Netherlands. If you haven't been, I highly recommend it. It's a theme park, very similar to Disneyland but a lot quirkier and older! Anyway, we went a few years ago in late winter when the UK was enjoying back-to-back storms. Of course, we couldn't predict that, but the journey home was horrendous. We were in an end cabin (it was the only five-birth cabin left when I booked - always book the middle if you can) and the storm was so fierce that we were awake half of the night rolling back and forth, back and forth. It felt like we were in a hammock!

THERE ARE SOME POSITIVES THOUGH!

⚓ Lots of open spaces to walk around. This includes shops, bars and even play areas!

⚓ Multiple choices of food and the option to bring your own. Whenever we have been on a ferry there has been a buffet-style restaurant, occasionally a second restaurant that serves more bar snacks and ordered meals, and a café that serves sandwiches, pizza and nibbles. We usually opt for the buffet for dinner and breakfast but it is pricey and we've decided that next time we would grab a McDonald's on the way down to the ferry for dinner and take some snacks on board.

⚓ It allows you to travel abroad and still take your car.

⚓ Entertainment is usually offered on board – there are cinemas and game rooms – but, if you have a cabin, you also have the option of your private space.

⚓ Usually more cost-effective than flying.

⚓ When it comes to a ferry, the security procedures aren't especially lengthy. In fact, in my experience they have been almost nonexistent. You can pack your car full and just tootle up to the boat and there is no worry about whether you will be allowed fluids or any of the faff you have with flying. They do check passports and tickets, which can lead to a long queue and wait times, but that is about it. You're also allowed to jump out of your car to soothe a baby if you're in the queue.

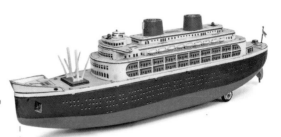

DRAWBACKS

⚓ The aforementioned rocky journey that can lead to seasickness in even the strongest stomach.

⚓ Takes longer than flying.

⚓ Limited to where you can go. You can't hop on a ferry and travel anywhere in the world as you are limited to certain ferry routes and you might well face a long drive before and/or after.

⚓ Can be a bit rowdy. Ferries are usually cost-effective so it's not uncommon to see big groups of people on celebration weekends, such as stag/hen dos or birthdays. It means it can get a little rowdy, especially in the bars or the casino (which you won't be frequenting with little ones but you may need to walk past). This has only been our experience once and I think it really depends on your destination of choice. I also don't think it's necessarily a bad thing, but possibly something to be aware of.

TRAVEL SICKNESS

Travel sickness is one of the most frustrating things as it's simply awful and it feels like there isn't much you can do about it. Sipping on cool water and nibbling on plain crackers or ginger biscuits can help. Try using a travel sickness wrist band. Worn before you set off, they use pressure points to try and relieve the symptoms. Sea-Band are well regarded and they do a variety of colours for adults and children.

If you have a different surname to your child, it is a wise idea to carry their birth certificate with you. I hadn't changed my surname to my married name on my passport and was asked, upon returning to the UK, to provide birth certificates or some additional identification to show that these were my children.

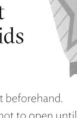
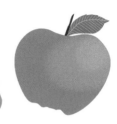

Getting the best out of travelling with kids on a ferry

⚓ Take snacks and book a meal or eat beforehand. Shops and restaurants on ferries tend not to open until the ship is far enough away from land to warrant being in 'open water', which means that, if you don't have any snacks with you, you can find yourself with hungry children for a few hours and only overpriced café food to keep them going.

⚓ Make sure you take everything out of your car that you will need, for that evening AND the following morning. I can't tell you how often I have forgotten something minor like, ahem, clothes for the next day so we have all had to wear the same outfits (regardless of how much food the kids have spilt down them at dinner!). Once you're upstairs, the crew won't let you back down unless someone can accompany you and they usually won't allow that unless it's for medicines or something urgent.

⚓ Give yourself plenty of time to get there. Final boarding will usually be 1–2 hours before the ship is due to set sale. However, you can board much earlier than this and we usually aim for 3–4 hours prior to sailing as that way you can have a look around, grab yourself a coffee and let the children have a play in the play area.

⚓ Check in online and have a look at the entertainment schedule. While you might not be drinking cocktails and joining in with the karaoke until 2 am, it's worth checking out the entertainment as there's often a show with Disney-based music early on and it can be much more family-orientated than you might assume. There is often a children's entertainer and disco and the cinemas show children's films early on too – but be aware that if you are watching a movie over the departure, it will be paused for the announcements and this takes at least 10–15 minutes.

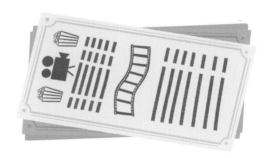

⚓ Queue early for dinner if you have booked it. On most ferries, the queue for the dining hall starts 20–30 minutes before it opens so I would suggest getting in it early to avoid a long wait before you get your seats.

⚓ Book breakfast, but get up early. If you've got children like mine who are up at the arse-crack of dawn and will want a breakfast relatively soon after they open their peepers, then book a breakfast. A lot of people don't bother to book, preferring the extra hour in bed, so the queues for the café are always filled with people seeking their morning coffee. If you're unsure about whether to book breakfast or dinner and don't want to book both, I would go with breakfast.

⚓ Ask about upgrading your room. This often only costs a little bit extra but it means you might end up with a LOT more space.

⚓ Book the best room you can, in the centre of the ship. Trust me, as I mentioned before, do your best to avoid the end or front rooms... or pack extra sickness tablets for the stormy weather.

P&O Ferries get my vote. We've travelled on a few ferries now and, without any doubt, P&O have always been my favourite. You do spend a little bit more but they are still very reasonably priced, the staff are invariably fabulous and hardworking and they have so many amenities and clean bedrooms. It's always a yes from me.

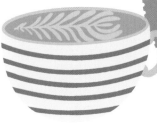

efteling, netherlands

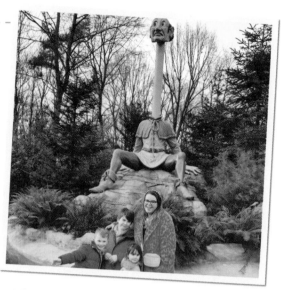

The word that instantly springs to mind to describe Efteling is 'quirky'. The first time we visited was for a press trip when they opened the Symbolica ride and the newest Loonsche Land holiday village. Like a lot of Brits, I'd never even heard of Efteling so I was going in as a complete newb and it blew my mind - so much so that we have been back again and the children talk about it all the time.

My favourite way of travelling to Efteling is by ferry. We load up the car, head to Hull (luckily for us, only 40 minutes away) and take the overnight ferry to Rotterdam, which is then only a 60–90 minute drive away from Efteling. I remember when I first drove off the ferry, I was so nervous that I wouldn't be any good at driving in another country, but it was totally fine! The children were in the back in their car seats spotting the long boats as we drove, marvelling at how level everything seemed and generally spotting things that they wouldn't normally see at home.

When you get close to Efteling, the first thing you see is the Efteling Hotel. I would love to stay there next time as it's a sight to behold and the kids love catching their first glimpse of it – an architectural gem that looks like it's floating in the air! Drive a little bit further and you arrive at the car park for day visitors (and if you're in the Netherlands and you have time it's worth that day visit), and then if you turn left and drive past the Efteling Hotel you come to the Loonsche Land village and hotel which is where we have stayed in the past. There are options to stay in the hotel, where the rooms have a really cool Scandi vibe, or self-catering holiday homes and we've tried both. I highly recommend the self-catering as there's pizza

delivery in case you don't fancy cooking yourself and a brilliant Lidl 0.7 miles down the road!

The food at Efteling hotels is quite limited and pricey. The continental breakfast at the hotel has a very narrow range of cereals and pastries and so self-catering can give you many more options. Or, if you're feeling flush and fancy, try the pancake house inside the Efteling park – it's really expensive but a wonderful experience and the pancakes are great. In self-catering, the kids also loved the beds! We had a large double bed with a ladder to the side that led up to two opposite-end loft beds – naturally they ALL had to sleep in loft beds, while Adam and I took the double bed in the second room.

As a guest at the parks, you get a little bit of extra time before day guests arrive, so once we had had our breakfast, we would head out early to make the most of all the attractions before the crowds flooded in. To the best of my knowledge, Efteling has no queue-jumping system, so I highly recommend planning your day and getting into the parks early. However, there are also so many things to see and do and that don't require any queuing at all!

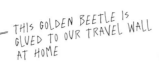

THIS GOLDEN BEETLE IS GLUED TO OUR TRAVEL WALL AT HOME

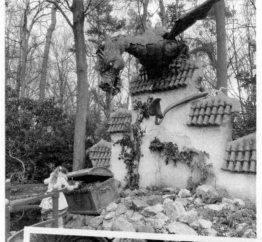

One of our favourite memories of Efteling is strolling around the Fairy tale forest for hours, looking at the weird and the wonderful ways in which they have brought fairy tales like Sleeping Beauty and Hansel and Gretel to life. Efteling, unlike the majority of theme parks aimed at families, seems to have retained a certain charm that hasn't been blighted by commercialisation. Yes, of course, there are loads of different shops and merchandise, but it isn't over the top or always in your face around the park.

I remember ordering one of the spiralled potatoes on a stick for everyone. Three suspicious pairs of eyes looked at me, questioning whether or not they should try this bizarre food. After much reassurance that this was really just a potato chopped up and sliced around a stick they gave it a go and it became a firm favourite with us all, coupled with a bottle of Chocomel or Chocomel hot chocolate.

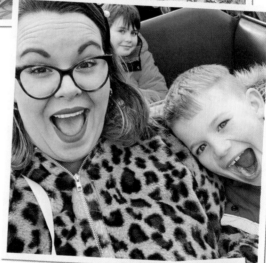

Efteling is the ideal place to visit via ferry with your car because, thanks to its central location, you can combine it with so much other great sightseeing. A long weekend at Efteling is plenty, but if you wanted to stop over for a bit longer, you could head into Rotterdam or Amsterdam. We visited the Blijdorp Zoo (Rotterdam Zoo) and had the best day out as their polar bear section was outstanding. It made a wonderful day trip, but if we had had a bit more time (and nicer weather) we could also have headed to the Plaswijckpark, which is a children's play park aimed at encouraging kids to run free and explore.

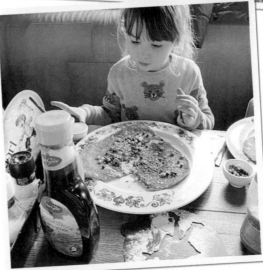

Travelling by plane

Arguably, this is the method of travel that the majority of us will use the least but worry about the most. Every day, thousands of parents search Google for 'tips for flying with children' or 'flying with a baby'. My own blog posts on the topics see a huge surge in popularity during holiday season, especially the ones about flying with babies. It is daunting. You can't exactly explain to a baby that they have to wait out a feed or convince a child mid-temper tantrum that they need to pipe down because they are disturbing everyone at 35,000 feet.

If you have never flown with a little one (especially a baby) before, it's perfectly reasonable to be scared about getting it all wrong and spending every second of the flight wishing that time would pass faster.

I've now reached the point where I'm not especially daunted by the thought of flying with my kids. In fact, I think I reached that point after Edith's first trip to Florida because it couldn't really have been any worse and yet the world didn't crumble when it was really hard, even though it felt like it a little at the time.

SO, WHAT ARE THE POSITIVES OF FLYING?

✈ You can basically go anywhere you like and fairly quickly.

✈ Toilets and food are all available on board, including proper meals, if you want them.

✈ Entertainment systems are usually built in, and if not, you will still be able to sit and enjoy your own entertainment.

✈ Lots of great, dedicated flight staff willing to help, just ask – we've only had the odd occasion where staff haven't been brilliant.

✈ Plenty of room to get up and move about, depending on the aircraft.

✈ Actually one of the safest methods of travel.

THE NOT SO GREAT?

✈ Airports, specifically the waiting around and security restrictions, are often considered one of the worst parts of flying. It can be stressful, but it doesn't have to be!

✈ Strict rules on what you can and can't have with you on board means you could be without something for hours.

✈ It's expensive.

✈ A lot of people are anxious about flying because it feels unnatural to be in the air.

✈ You're in a confined space and there is no option to leave if your kids are kicking off.

✈ Jet lag. It's a bitch.

WHAT TO INCLUDE IN A CHILD'S HAND LUGGAGE/FOR THEM IN YOURS

- ☐ Snacks, not overly sugary
- ☐ Drinks beaker (if needed)
- ☐ Pre-loaded tablet or device like Nintendo 3DS, if they have one
- ☐ Colouring pads
- ☐ Colouring pencils – we avoided felt tips when they were tiny
- ☐ Wipes
- ☐ Reusable sticker books (Melissa & Doug books are fabulous)
- ☐ Story book for reading
- ☐ Favourite teddy/comforter
- ☐ We buy some inexpensive mini toys like blind bags and pull one out every time the kids seem to be getting a bit bored on long-haul flights. It helps keep them entertained and they love the surprise.
- ☐ Headphones (they are comfier/ better than the ones you get on board)
- ☐ Something like Lego or even the aqua beads sets that require concentration and keep them busy.

How to get the best out of flying

✈ Arrive early. Airport arrivals vary, depending on whether you are flying internationally or not. I'm that person who likes to arrive super early and have breakfast/lunch/dinner and a mooch around the duty free. That way, I'm always through security and ready-to-roll way before I need to be.

✈ If you're flying with children or a baby, they usually get a luggage and hand luggage allowance too, so pack a bag. My children have had their own hand luggage since they were old enough to carry a bag. Even if it is only a tiny bag or backpack, it's enough for them to carry their tablets, colouring pencils and books and a teddy. Yes, I'm overall responsible for them not forgetting/leaving the bag somewhere, but it takes the pressure off me.

✈ Check with your airline about what you're allowed as a 'free item' for your baby. It's usually a car seat OR a pushchair, but double check beforehand that you won't have to pay extra.

✈ You can take empty sippy cups on board if you're worried about your child spilling. However, don't fill them unless there is a medical reason (you will likely need a doctor's note that has been pre-authorised).

✈ Don't forget to check on VISAs and whether you need them, at least a week before travel.

✈ For a baby, you are allowed to pack formula and/or expressed breastmilk. Up until recently, the rules were that you would be asked to test the milk or you would be told no, if it was over a certain limit. However, the advice is always subject to change and I recommend that you check the information about hand luggage restrictions before you set off. At the moment, you can take a 'reasonable' amount of pre-made formula or sterilised water and powder onto the aircraft and up to 2000ml breast milk in individual containers. That is A LOT. You can also take cool gel packs and bags, soya milk and baby food. Frozen breast milk needs to be in the hold. For most of this, you will be expected to have the baby with you and that's it.

✈ Take a small bag with you that you can wear across your body to contain your phone, tickets and passports. I only worked this out recently and it was a LIFE SAVER! I carry a little bag by Vooray called a 'Sidekick' and it's fantastic for travelling. I wear it across my body, underneath coats and I don't have to delve into all the many pockets of huge travel bags or worry that I've lost what I need. I then save the big ole bag for kid's stuff.

✈ Pre-load tablets with games and download movies or TV series as wifi isn't strong enough and pricey on board.

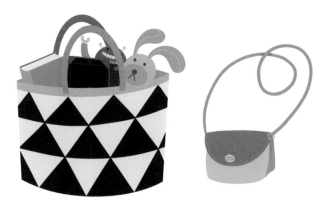

✈ Pre-book seats – it's not worth the trauma. I have a firm belief that, while flights operate the way they do, you need to book seats until legislation comes in and says 'stop being dickheads' to airlines that are monetising seat bookings. It IS true that an airline has an obligation to sit a child with a parent, and a lot of well known airlines will make sure that any child under 12 is sat with one parent, but you aren't able to guarantee all of you sat together, and sat with a parent can mean in front of you, to the side of you and one line removed. My kids would be hysterical if we were separated, so I always factor seat booking into my holiday cost.

✈ Extra leg room seats are worth it with a toddler or crawler during long-haul flights and sometimes even with older kids. When we flew to Florida with a tiny Edith, it was the first time Adam had flown for 11 hours, so I paid the extra and booked the seats with leg room. Edith sat at my feet for a part of the journey and played happily with little toys. I did eventually have to pick her up and carry her up and down the plane, mind, but it was such a good thing while it lasted.

✈ Pre-book children's meals and vegetarian meals. If you don't pre-book 'special requirements', you will get the standard offering and that isn't always great for children, never mind the picky ones.

✈ You can pre-book to be fast-tracked through security – but check your airport policy because you often don't have to pay to use the fast track if you have young children or a member of your party is disabled. This also applies to those with large items such as car seats and/or pushchairs.

✈ Charger packs are your friends – grab a double charger that will charge for as long as you need it.

✈ Baby food pouches can be ordered in bulk from places like boots.com and shipped to your hotel of choice, if you feel you need them.

✈ If you're going somewhere where you think you're going to be doing a lot of shopping and bringing more home, then either lightly pack a suitcase or pack a suitcase inside another suitcase, as that way you won't have to buy another on the way home.

Simply for Flying is a wonderful company that makes little flight log books for children to record their flight experiences. We bought three when the children were tiny (before Edith was born actually!) and, every time we fly, be it long- or short-haul, we ask a flight attendant to get the Captain to fill in the book. It's such a small thing but it's wonderful to look back at and, every time we fly, I'm asked by the staff where they can get one for their own kids. There is even a little place to pop tickets too! https://simplyforflying.com

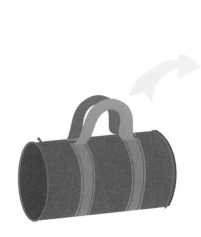

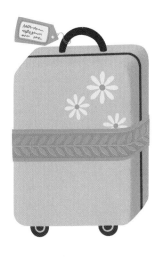

Travel bucket list

I'm a big believer in the power of willing something into existence. It might take you a long time, it might be a really hard slog, but I firmly believe in actualising your dreams. If your dreams are to travel, then here is your place to jot them down.

'Two of the greatest gifts we can give our children are roots and wings.'
HODDING CARTER

Travelling abroad

In my experience, travelling abroad with your children is one of the most amazing things you can do. It's never 'not worth it'. Regardless of their age, there will always be a memory that you will treasure forever and, as they grow, there will be memories that they will hold on to too. I still remember travelling to Spain with my mum when I was a kid. We didn't have a lot of money. My mum was a single mother on a nurse's wage, so we would save up for flights and then a friend would let us stay in their villa. Some of my dearest memories are from those weeks when we'd lie out on the sundeck, relaxing with our feet up and mum reading to me. I could only have been seven or eight years old, but the memories have stuck. During my teenage years we didn't really travel at all. We didn't have the money and the villa had been sold. Now, as an adult and mother myself, taking our own children away, or going away for a weekend of reconnecting and discovering new things with my husband, has filled the memory banks with the most joyful moments, both mine and theirs.

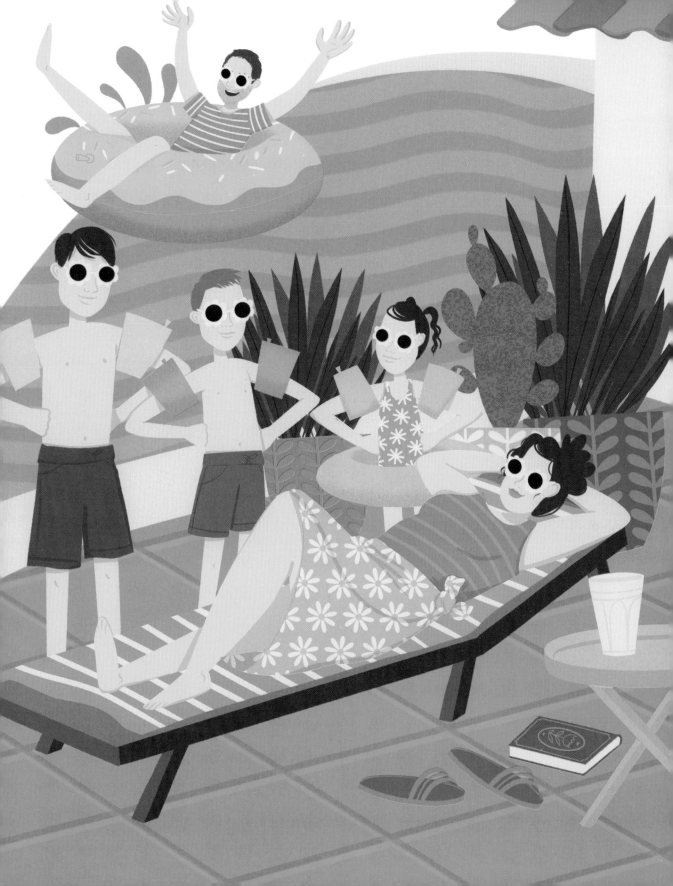

Mum's suitcase checklist

One of the things I'm asked most frequently about travelling abroad is what to pack on holiday with babies and children.
I am a self-confessed list-maker. When we are travelling, I have a list for everyone in the family (including my husband's stuff...) because organisation is the key to avoiding insanity when it comes to travelling with kids. To spare my non-list-making readers, I've popped together a checklist of the things that I would take abroad with me, from birth to adulthood.

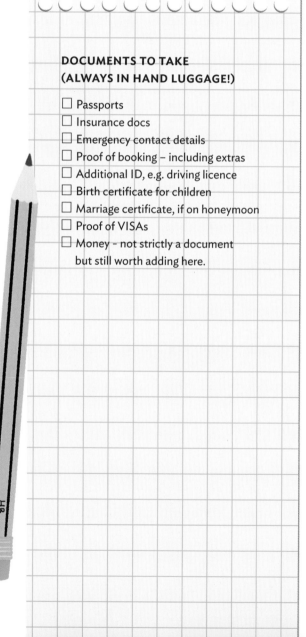

DOCUMENTS TO TAKE
(ALWAYS IN HAND LUGGAGE!)

☐ Passports
☐ Insurance docs
☐ Emergency contact details
☐ Proof of booking – including extras
☐ Additional ID, e.g. driving licence
☐ Birth certificate for children
☐ Marriage certificate, if on honeymoon
☐ Proof of VISAs
☐ Money - not strictly a document but still worth adding here.

BABIES AND TODDLERS UNDER 2 (7 DAY HOLIDAY)

- [ ] Nappies (you can buy these in airports and abroad but, if you have a little one that is sensitive to nappy rash or you don't want to spend a fortune on branded nappies, I would take them with you)
- [ ] Baby food, if required (you can have it sent out too, remember)
- [ ] 3–4 feeding bottles, if required
- [ ] Travel steriliser and equipment, if required (often fairly small and easy to fit in a case)
- [ ] Travel breast pump, if you want to express
- [ ] Breast pads (obviously not for the baby but worth adding here; reusable ones are good for travelling because you can rinse them and reuse so they take up less space)
- [ ] An easy-fold, lie-flat pushchair
- [ ] 2–3 large muslin squares for keeping cool/using as a blanket (or, if you want, you can use them as a breastfeeding cover – in some countries this is advisable but, in most places in my experience, people are disinterested in a baby having a meal)
- [ ] Wet wipes (or cloths)
- [ ] Nappy cream
- [ ] Baby sunscreen
- [ ] Swim nappies
- [ ] Medication (like Calpol)
- [ ] 4–5 baby/toddler outfits (I never pack one for every day; kids just don't care if they re-wear clothes and you will have less washing to do when you get back!)
- [ ] 2 baby/toddler swimwear outfits
- [ ] 4–5 baby/toddler sleepsuits/PJs
- [ ] Baby sunglasses and hat
- [ ] Socks/a pair of comfy shoes for walkers. Avoid jelly shoes in heat.

NON-ESSENTIALS BUT WORTH CONSIDERING

- [ ] Car seat (essential for a car, not public transport)
- [ ] Swim seat/float
- [ ] Foldable baby tent to avoid sun
- [ ] Pushchair cover (be careful to ensure it's breathable and safe) or parasol.

EVERYONE ELSE (7 DAY HOLIDAY)

- [ ] Medication and first aid kit to include plasters (include some blister plasters in here – they are amazing)
- [ ] Sun cream/aftersun
- [ ] 2 x swimwear
- [ ] 4–5 T-shirts and/or dresses (take more for teens/adults if you like options)
- [ ] 3 shorts or skirts (take more for teens/adults if you like options)
- [ ] 2–3 smarter outfits (take more if you feel you need it)
- [ ] Sunglasses and hat
- [ ] 1–2 pair(s) shoes/sandals (avoid jelly shoes)
- [ ] Chargers/charging wires
- [ ] Make-up kit and remover
- [ ] Deodorant and perfume (place in a waterproof bag or buy new as aerosol products and perfumes can leak due to air pressure)
- [ ] Body wash and shampoo
- [ ] Hair curlers or straighteners if you want them
- [ ] Bug spray, if required
- [ ] 2–3 PJs
- [ ] Any jewellery you wish to take

cascais, portugal

One of my favourite places in the world is Cascais in Portugal. We have only been once but it has a really special place in my heart and I just love it. I often joke to Adam that, one day, we're going to own a house there and eat cheese with honey and nuts to our hearts' content.

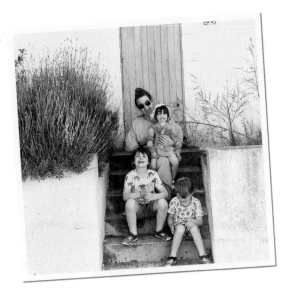

We went to Cascais for the first time when the children were tiny, as part of a work trip. We stayed just outside the town, up in the hills at a place called the Martinhal Resort (lovely and family-friendly, but it's pricey), so we had to get a bus into the town. We'd then walk down beautiful cobbled streets, past markets and all the lovely restaurants serving fresh seafood, through the central square, where you could buy the most wonderful ice cream, and then sit on the Praia da Ribeira beach. It's tiny so often really crowded, but the crystal clear water is full of little fish and it overlooks the harbour.

If you want a proper beach that you can lounge on and watch the kids play for hours, Cascais is surrounded by gorgeous coastline, and the beach Praia da Conceição is really easy to get to (walking distance) and just beautiful. One of the things I really regret not going to see, and I think it's because we had the children with us and the trip wasn't 'pushchair friendly', is the magnificent Pena Palace which is set up in the hills of Serra de Sintra (Serra de Sintra also has a host of beaches for the more wild at heart, perhaps with older children/teens who love surfing). When we head back, it's high on the agenda!

And you can also visit Lisbon as it's only a 40-minute train journey away. We stayed at the Lisbon Martinhal hotel and it was fabulous. And for me the highlight of the city was the Oceanário de Lisboa (Lisbon Aquarium). If you are staying in Cascais then I highly recommend it for a day visit as it was spectacular. Make sure you pause as you walk up the ramps to watch the jellyfish in the water below, a very unexpected bonus for us! The Sao Jorge castle was a beautiful day out too, especially for free-range kids looking for something more than the beach and cobbled streets of Cascais. There is just so much to see and the café does lovely cakes too.

When you're walking around Cascais (or Lisbon) there are lots of incredible market stalls. If you like to bring craft or artworks or jewellery home, then I highly recommend them.

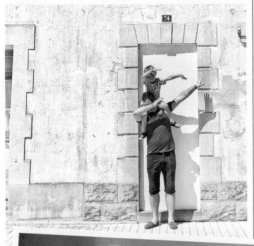

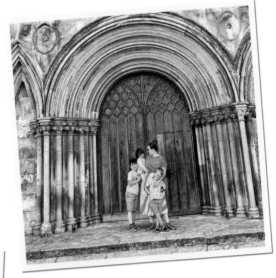

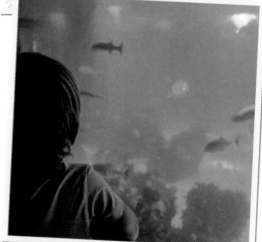

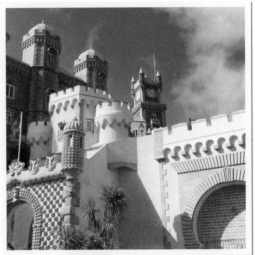

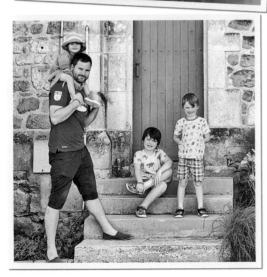

PENA PALACE OUTSIDE
LISBON, FOR NEXT TIME...

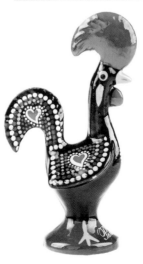

Making a scrap book or memory box

One of my favourite things to do when we have been on holiday is to create a scrapbook or memory box for the kids. I think it all began when I was younger and my mum took me to Miami to see some friends as the shop next to their gym was a scrapbook and crafting shop, something we didn't really have in the UK at the time, and I filled up a scrapbook with all my precious things from our holiday.

I like to use a box – it's simple and, quite frankly, requires much less effort than a beautifully decorated book. If I throw in my strange collection of memorable items from the holiday, I know that, years from now, the kids will be able to delve into all the things I've kept for them and experience a warm rush of memories.

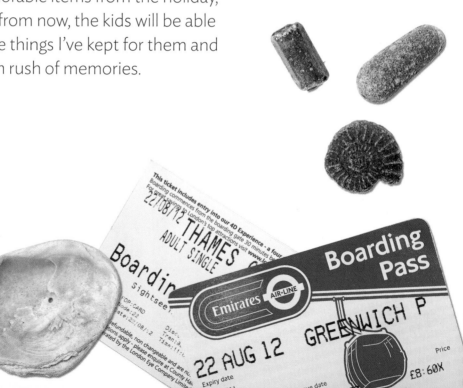

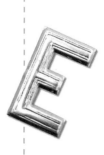

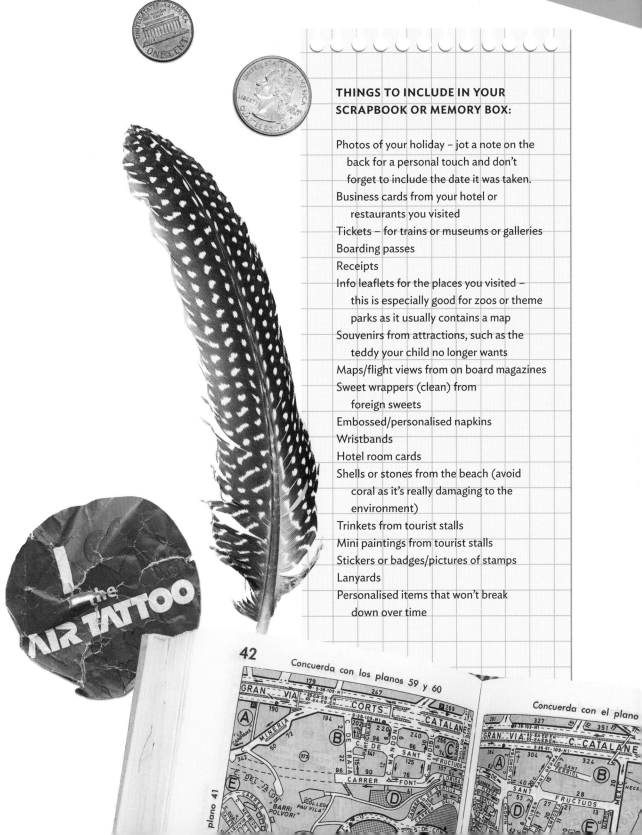

THINGS TO INCLUDE IN YOUR SCRAPBOOK OR MEMORY BOX:

Photos of your holiday – jot a note on the
    back for a personal touch and don't
    forget to include the date it was taken.
Business cards from your hotel or
    restaurants you visited
Tickets – for trains or museums or galleries
Boarding passes
Receipts
Info leaflets for the places you visited –
    this is especially good for zoos or theme
    parks as it usually contains a map
Souvenirs from attractions, such as the
    teddy your child no longer wants
Maps/flight views from on board magazines
Sweet wrappers (clean) from
    foreign sweets
Embossed/personalised napkins
Wristbands
Hotel room cards
Shells or stones from the beach (avoid
    coral as it's really damaging to the
    environment)
Trinkets from tourist stalls
Mini paintings from tourist stalls
Stickers or badges/pictures of stamps
Lanyards
Personalised items that won't break
    down over time

42

Travel and education

The world is an amazing classroom and travelling is the ultimate teacher. There are so many amazing places to see, some obviously educational, like a museum or historical building, but others less obvious and equally important.

I think that everything you do abroad is a way of learning about a new culture. It's for this reason that we have happily taken the children out of school when we have felt it is appropriate, avoiding the busy crowds and extra cost that comes with the school holidays. I would encourage you not to dismiss term time just because it might cost you a fine. At the time of writing, you can be fined for removing your child from school unless your head teacher gives permission. What this means is that you will receive a letter from your local authority telling you that your child has been absent without permission ('unauthorised absence') and you are required to pay a fine per child. Sometimes, you will have an 'unauthorised absence' but receive no letter. It all depends on whether your child has a certain amount of absent days already, even if these are for illness or, as in our case with Toby, a potentially life-saving operation. Ultimately though, no one can stop you taking your child on holiday.

LET'S GET EDUCATING!

If you are taking your child out of school to go on holiday then they will have the bonus of learning about travel and culture, but sometimes you have to weigh up whether or not they will be missing something crucial at school that might help them, how long they will be missing and what they will need to catch up on. Teachers are highly unlikely to have the time to help your child catch up if they have missed out on work.

ASK YOUR TEACHER FOR ADVICE ON WHERE YOUR CHILD IS ON THE CURRICULUM

I usually ask our teacher what their plan will be for the next couple of weeks and try to encourage my kids to do certain things while we're travelling or while we're having some relaxing time at the hotel. One year, Reuben's teacher really kindly printed off a load of extra bits for him to do, but I would never expect this as teachers already have so much work. You can find a million and one resources online. Places like twinkl. co.uk have free resources for all ages, or you can type in 'free resources *insert child's year group or key stage*' and loads of things will come up. Pinterest is also a great place to find age-appropriate travel learning ideas. Alternatively, you could ask your teacher to set aside the worksheets and work that is printed at school during the days your child is absent and then catch up at home.

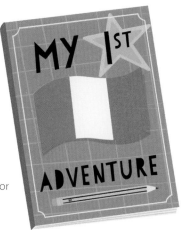

KEEP A JOURNAL

This is a great way to get children to practise their reading, writing, storytelling and information recall. You can stick in loads of photos or even use it as a scrapbook!

WORKBOOKS FOR ENTERTAINMENT ON THE PLANE

I know, it doesn't sound all that fun does it? But when you have next to nothing to do for hours on end, cracking out a workbook can be a great way to bust the boredom, especially if it's a themed one. Things like 'paint by numbers' are great for younger ones and you can even make your own – buy a really simple colouring book and add some maths equations (2+2, etc.) to each section, then use the answer for the code. This really helped Toby's times tables when we had a brief stint of home-educating during the coronavirus lockdown.

DON'T STRESS, COUNT ON THE GO AND ASK THEM TO REMEMBER ONE INTERESTING FACT THEY HAVE LEARNT EACH DAY

Life is learning. That's not a corny saying, it's true. Count the pink suitcases in the airport, read the signs, take advantage of the activity centres in the hotel or at a place that you visit, let your child use a camera to take pictures and then label them when they are home. There are so many things you can do and, ultimately, two weeks is not going to be the end of the world.

City breaks with kids

In my experience, city breaks are often considered purely for adults and something that would bore children silly. They want to 'play in a pool, run about at the beach or visit a child-themed attraction like Disneyworld' but this is SUCH a common misconception and cities have so much to offer kids.

> City breaks with kids are a totally different ball game to ones with just your partner or friends, so forget everything you might think of as a classic city break and change your mindset.

DO A BIT OF RESEARCH ON THE CITY YOU'RE VISITING

For every holiday destination there will be hundreds of blog posts, travel reviews and holiday sites to help you make the most of your trip. You are of course 'the expert' on your own child(ren), so combine this with the knowledge you have of your kids and you should have an idea of what will work. When we visit London, I read up on what is recommended and work out what would be age-appropriate: some of the museums just wouldn't be any fun for the kids and others are ideal. We have done the same around the world and every time we have found a gem that the kids have loved.

EXPECT IT TO BE TIRING

City breaks often involve a lot of walking and sightseeing and not a lot of resting. It's fairly tiring, so bear that in mind. TOP TIP: Start the day early and end it early. In my opinion, cities at night are always a bit meh for kids.

PICK A TOPIC TO LEARN ABOUT OR TO DISCOVER WHILST YOU ARE THERE

If you're visiting a city like Rome you could easily learn all about the Roman era, visit the ruins, the Colosseum and talk about being a gladiator. Or perhaps you're visiting Amsterdam and you could learn about the system of canals and go for a bike ride around the park (they are really cheap to rent, just make sure you grab yourself a cone of chips with peanut sauce afterwards).

ASK FOR TIPS

If you have social media, asking for tips from Facebook groups or your friends can be incredibly helpful. People might be able to share blog posts, links to recommendations on Trip advisor or even websites where you can pre-buy tickets. I would recommend buying tickets in advance for most places and planning out a rough itinerary for your break, just so you have an idea of where you're going and when.

HEAD OUT OF THE CITY IF YOU WANT TO

If you discover something outside of the city that is of interest, head out to it. About a 90-minute drive out of Barcelona is one of Spain's most famous theme parks, PortAventura. You can either stay over or just visit for the day – they even have a brilliant water park. Don't feel trapped in one place. You can leave the city and explore too.

jet lag

Jet lag is the ultimate pain in the arse with children and one of the most negative parts of travel. The best ways to avoid/handle jet lag are:

✈ Try to book a flight that allows you to sleep whilst it is night at your destination so you arrive with a good few hours of daylight to be had.

✈ Window seats can help you sleep on a flight.

✈ Avoid the booze and caffeine whilst on board and drink water or juice instead. (Ha, I know, I ignore that advice too!)

✈ Eat light, try not to eat anything too heavy.

✈ Try to get outside and explore when you arrive at your destination.

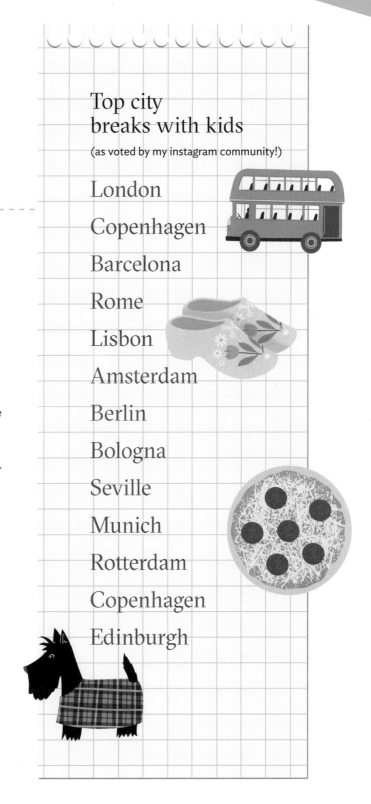

Top city breaks with kids

(as voted by my instagram community!)

London

Copenhagen

Barcelona

Rome

Lisbon

Amsterdam

Berlin

Bologna

Seville

Munich

Rotterdam

Copenhagen

Edinburgh

new york, new york

New York isn't necessarily somewhere you think of taking children, or it wasn't for me until last year. However, just after the New Year, during the Christmas school break, we travelled to New York as part of a work trip. The overwhelming advice I had from people was to avoid it with the children... but they couldn't have been more wrong. We had the BEST time! New York has a wealth of culture and history, not to mention loads of things for people of all ages.

When you arrive at JFK airport, you are not in for a treat. Unfortunately, it is, hands down, the worst airport I have visited in the world – disorganised and overcrowded BUT there is a way to avoid it all. If you fly from England to Dublin, with a connecting flight to New York, you can do all of the passport control stuff when you arrive in Dublin (super quick and easy) and then you simply fly through JFK. Of course, I didn't know this until it was too late, but I costed it up when we came home and the price really wasn't that different and would have spared us three horrible hours in customs. If you opt not to go through the connection route, then make sure you save some water from the plane for the queue. Use the toilet before you get off the plane and keep your kids' tablets at the ready –you're likely to need them.

Once you're out of the airport, the fun begins. We stayed right in the centre of Manhattan so we had easy access to the more touristy things. As you can imagine, this is where the majority of hotels are, but there are also some wonderful things across the Brooklyn Bridge around the Dumbo area that will afford you the most magical skyline view, so it's worth weighing up your options.

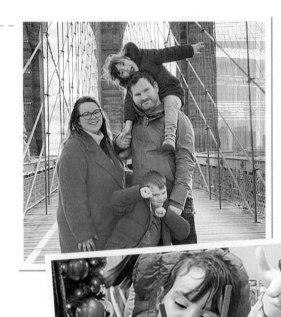

On our first evening in New York we visited Times Square. The children were mesmerised by the bright lights and the Disney characters – just don't let them jump on you for a photo as it will cost anywhere between $30 and 100 and they won't tell you until you have already taken the photo, so just look on from afar. If you've got a Marvel fan like we do, then just around the corner from Times Square is a little pizzeria called Joe's Pizza, which was featured in *Spiderman*. Of course, it's completely overpriced but it lit up Reuben's little face to see it. And then after taking in the bright lights, grabbing some pizza and looking in some of the major shops, we headed back to our hotel (which was right next to Grand Central station, which is well worth a visit and, for little ones, also the setting for parts of *Madagascar*) for an early night. The best piece of advice I had about New York with children was to start early and finish early.

The following morning, we woke up at 5:30 am (I'll take jet lag for 5 please Alex) and headed out to Ellen's Stardust diner. If you arrive after 7:30 am, be prepared to queue for ages, but get there early and you walk right in. It's like a lot of famous places in New York – overpriced as hell – but fantastic for the children who loved watching the servers jump up onto the tables to sing their hearts out. After a leisurely breakfast, we made a slow walk to the Rockefeller Center area, visited some of the amazing shops like FAO Schwartz (get there early enough and you can play the famous piano from *Big*), the American Girl store for Edith and watched the ice skaters. We waited until the evening to visit the Top of the Rock because it's beautiful at night. It takes around 45 minutes to get up to the top, so be aware that your kids will be queuing for that long, or head across to one of the other skylines that are less well known.

The following day we headed to the Trolls Experience. While it was pricey, it was no more than the usual family attraction and the children got a Trolls makeover, played games and were well and truly exhausted by the time we were finished. We headed into Central Park and took a horse and carriage ride – personally, next time I would just enjoy walking around, grabbing snacks from the street vendors and visiting the zoo. The carriage ride was lovely, but it was dark and we couldn't see a lot of the things that were being pointed out. Central Park Zoo was a lovely little walk around and the kids adored watching the sea lions jumping about. They have a restaurant inside,

but the prices are steep and you're much better off eating before you go in and then grabbing something on the way out. Pretzels are always a good shout! One of the best things about New York is that, for a city nicknamed the Concrete Jungle, it's amazing how many green spaces there are, which are ideal for sitting down and resting your feet. If you fancy trying something eccentric after your morning in Central Park, head to Dylan's Candy Bar, an amazing sweet shop, and then up the street to Serendipity for their iced hot chocolate. It's glorious, and the food was really yummy too! Just be aware that, like with everything in New York, it's expensive and you will need to leave a tip.

Visiting DUMBO was the highlight of my whole trip. Who knew that watching the children running across the Brooklyn Bridge (a 35-40 minute walk and pushchair friendly) would be so wonderful? But they absolutely loved it and the views are so worth it. When you get across, spend time walking about. There are some great little play areas and lovely independent shops that are a far cry from the touristy vibe of Manhattan. For lunch, head to the Time Out Market – make sure you grab some cookie dough – and then walk up to the top of the building to look around. It gets fairly busy, so try to go for an early lunch around 11:30 am.

New York exceeded our expectations as a family. We might have come home exhausted and having walked our little feet off, but it was such fun. It reminded us that concrete jungles can be just as fun as the beaches and pools that we have come to associate with family travel.

WE BOUGHT CHRISTMAS TREE DECS TO REMIND US

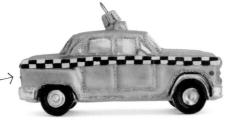

Staycationing*

When my mum was a little girl, travel wasn't that easy. It wasn't a case of just hopping on a plane – she had nine siblings and her father was a miner. Travel wasn't exactly a priority when it was hard enough putting food on the table. However, while flights to the unknown were fairly uncommon, staycationing (though it was never called that, it was *just* a holiday) was the norm. Seaside holidays were the ultimate joy. We have such beautiful coastal areas here in the UK and yet often we don't think of going there as 'a real holiday'.

However, staycationing is making a welcome comeback, and it's something that I have learnt to really love. When Reuben was tiny, I remember saying to Adam that it doesn't really count as a proper holiday if we aren't going abroad, yet now I realise how ridiculous that sounds. After all, some of my very best memories have been had at Center Parcs' holiday complexes, or surfing in the Cornish sea. I've been lucky enough to staycation with my family up and down the country as well as travel abroad and I can say with complete faith that staycationing has so much to offer and, when you're weighing up holiday options, you really shouldn't dismiss it.

* STAYCATION
A staycation, or holistay, (portmanteau of 'stay' and 'vacation', 'holiday' and 'stay') is a period when an individual or family goes on holiday without going abroad.

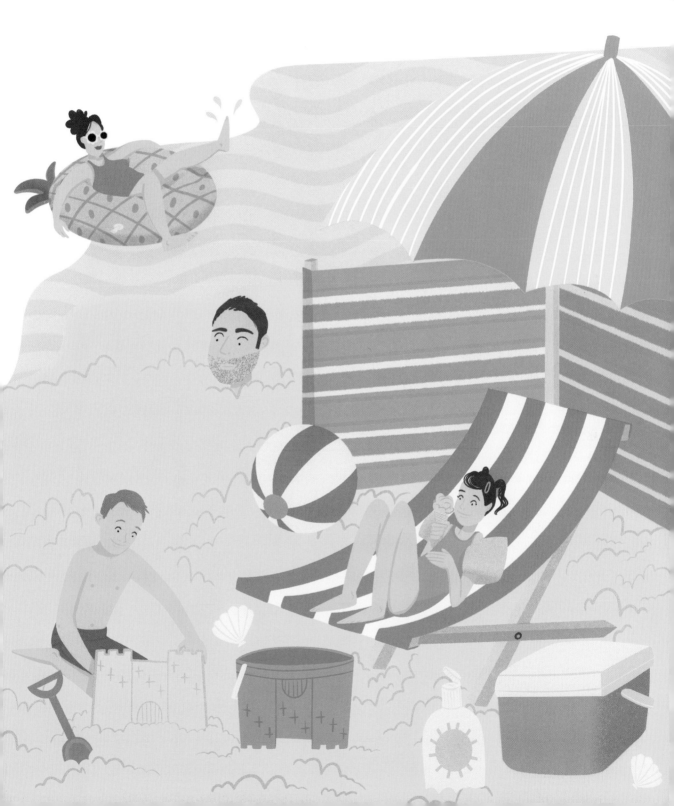

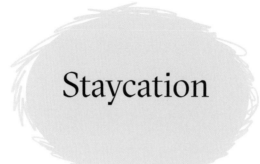

Staycation

Pros

You can take anything you want with you, often including pets.

You know what kind of shops and amenities you will get – no second guessing if you will be able to buy nappies or baby food.

Everything can be reached by car or public transport.

You don't have to worry about passports and VISAs.

It is usually much more economical than travelling abroad.

It is better for the environment.

You can see/learn about your own heritage and country.

The travel rating system will usually be in line with what Brits expect – 5* will mean 5*.

It is often easier to do as a large group or family because you can rent a house/cottage.

There will be no jet lag/time zone woes (especially helpful with children).

Cons

The weather isn't always great – though there really is no guarantee of weather anywhere in the world, we are an especially rainy/grey country at times.

It's a little limited in terms of cultural experience – it's too familiar.

Sightseeing is more limited – you may well have seen a lot of the sights that are available near to where you are staying.

While you can access the places you want to go in a car or via public transport, it frequently takes a long time. For us, living in the North of England, travelling to Cornwall was a 9 ½ hour trip. We could have flown to tourist hotspots in Europe… and back.

It can be more expensive than you think – while the travelling element is undoubtably less expensive, I've found that it's not all that much cheaper to staycation if you're eating out and visiting heritage sites or paid-for attractions.

Vacation ← OR HOLIDAY BECAUSE, YOU KNOW, BRITISH

Pros

Travelling to other countries means experiencing other cultures firsthand.

There is more chance of hot sunny weather if you choose the right spot.

You'll see firsthand things that you might otherwise only see in books.

You will enjoy the enriching experience of foreign travel in general.

Seeing the world is such a privilege – if you have the opportunity, it is worth doing.

It's an educational experience, and you might have the opportunity to practise languages that your children are learning at school.

Cons

There is the environmental impact (you can offset this if you are of a mind to – there are many websites where you can calculate the impact of your journey and pay a fee to plant however many trees would be needed to offset the carbon emissions of your trip.

Depending on your family set-up, you may need to consider the laws of the country. As a white, heterosexual married couple this is something that has never impacted myself and my husband, but after chatting to friends who have a different family set-up, it's often a consideration for them.

You can't just take EVERYTHING with you, though you can take a lot.

Forget something? Chances are you might not be able to get the exact brand of nappy or food your child likes and, depending on your child (particularly if they have special needs), that might be an issue to consider.

It can be very expensive.

You need to remember to take important documents with you and it can be a pain if you lose them.

How to get the best out of a staycation

So, you've weighed it up and come to the conclusion that a staycation is for you, but where to begin? Staycationing is exactly the same as going abroad in that there are so many ways to do it, from the private holiday home (think villa-style) to the opposite end of the spectrum that is the holiday complex.

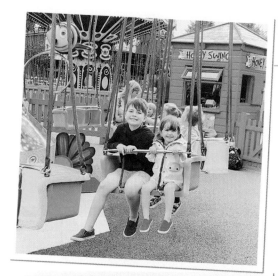

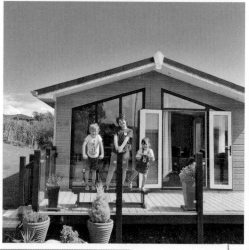

WORK OUT WHAT YOU WANT, THEN PLAN

When it comes to planning a staycation, I usually start with working out what kind of holiday I'm after. Do I want to sightsee or head to the beach? Am I going to be out all the time or do I want to stay on a complex that will give me everything I want so I won't need to leave? Will this be during term time in the summer, when everything is a little cheaper, or during the holidays in the winter, when my options will be fairly limited?

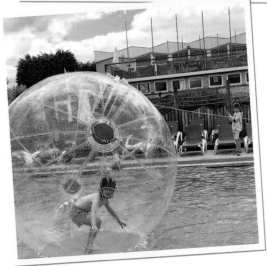

What are the options?

HOLIDAY COMPLEXES WHERE YOU STAY AND DON'T REALLY LEAVE

Places like Center Parcs are ideal for small families who want to essentially have a complete holiday without much travel. There is a pool (indoor and warm all year which makes it easy to forget you are in the UK if it's bucketing it down), restaurants, shops and a host of options should you wish to self-cater. There are options to suit almost all budgets, with varying degrees of luxury, from a simple lodge where you bring everything (including your toilet paper!) to a lodge with maid service, hot tub and games room. Activities are plentiful too, you just have to pay for them. In my experience, as someone who has stayed at Center Parcs frequently, they aren't so keen on you coming and going. You can, but you need to find someone to let you in and out, and with it being more expensive to stay on this kind of complex with secure car parks and locked gates than in something like a Haven or Butlins where you're expected to come and go, it begs the question why you would pay extra to head off site instead of staying and using the facilities.

HOLIDAY COMPLEXES WHERE YOU CAN COME AND GO BUT THAT STILL OFFER RESTAURANTS, SHOPS AND ENTERTAINMENT AND SELF-CATERING ACCOMMODATION (USUALLY CARAVAN OR STATIC HOMES)

Places like Haven, Butlins or independent caravan parks are perfect if you are looking for a self-catering complex where you can come and go, usually near a beach location and surrounded by historical sites. I love this kind of holiday – there are usually pools and activities that you can book but the expectation is that you will come and go from the complex a bit.

THEME PARK HOLIDAYS

Places like Chessington World of Adventures, Legoland or similar are great if you have children who love rides or just love theme parks in general. You can usually book long-weekend stays. Food is sometimes included, depending on prices, and the park tickets are included too. They often host seasonal events too when the prices are much cheaper but when only select things are open.

HOTELS OR B&BS WITH ROOMS

A hotel can be great and provide the most opportunity for relaxation. However, it does also mean that you're limited to the space of one room and often there is no catering beyond tea- and coffee-making facilities. We have stayed in hotels up and down the country for one-night stays or long weekends and they are perfect for that and for city breaks or if you want to get close to a specific destination, but often not ideal for more than two to three days. Also, as a large family, hotels cost us a huge amount of money because we need a suite or two rooms. A real pain in the arse!

A PRIVATE HOLIDAY COTTAGE OR APARTMENT

Great for large parties or if you want to travel somewhere and be totally flexible. It's the home away from home in a lot of cases and, while often a little pricier than a holiday park, you will have everything you need. However, you also ideally need a car, or you need to know the local taxi services and exactly how far you are from places you might want to visit. As obvious as it might sound, asking the who, what, where and when is the first thing to do before you book anywhere.

Check out the area you are staying

Regardless of where you choose to go, there are always things to see in the UK. It's so filled with historical sites and amazing views, be they the Yorkshire Wolds or the cliffs in Dorset, Stonehenge or Holyrood Palace. When you decide on an area and you choose your type of accommodation, check out English Heritage, National Trust and local tourism boards to see what is available in the area. There will be so much to discover! When we stayed just outside Torquay, we visited some really well-known places, like The Eden Project (amazing day out if you fancy it) but also some great hidden gems like the Torquay Dinosaur World, which delighted the children (and the fish and chip restaurant next door delighted me even more!).

Unpredictable weather

Unfortunately the weather can have a mind of it's own - we can have glorious sunshine one day and torrential rain the next, it's anyone's guess! Be prepared. We once took a lovely trip to Devon which had a glorious, sunny forecast, only for it to be bucketing it down and chilly. I hadn't packed anyone any cardigans or jumpers, just thin summer jackets... queue a trip to Tesco to try and grab something vaguely warm!

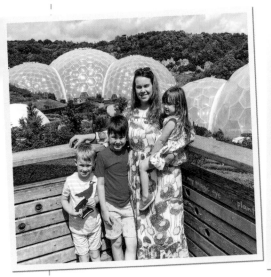

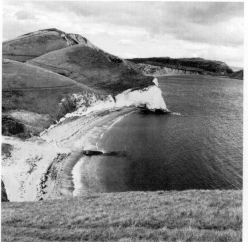

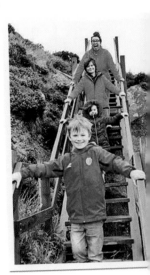

Take it all or spend it all

Depending on what you've chosen to do, there will be the question of what to do about food! Do you shop before you go and take it all with you, or buy it when you arrive or simply eat out every day? Places like Center Parcs or even a holiday park with static homes like Haven, make all options really easy and you can tailor it to your own needs. However, it becomes a bit more challenging when you're staying in a hotel or B&B. If you do decide to take everything with you, think about how long it will take you to get there (do you need a cool box?) and space in the car.

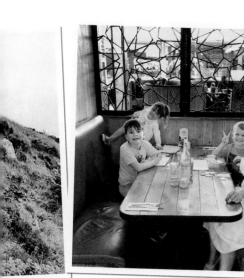

Staycation food checklist

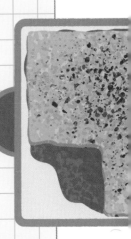

MEALS TO MAKE IN ADVANCE:
Good ole lasagne
Fresh Pizza to freeze
Casseroles
Curries (minus the rice)
Soups
Chilli con carne
Tagines
Bolognese
Stews
Pies (cooked, ready to reheat)
Shepherd or cottage pie

READY TO COOK WITH/ESSENTIALS
Vegetables of your choice
    (prepped veg are ideal for staycations)
Fruit of your choice
Rice
Pasta
Cereal
Butter
Oil
Milk
Bread
Any snacks you enjoy
Tea/coffee as this isn't always present
Sugar/sweetener
Alcohol or soft drinks

devon and cornwall

In the summer of 2018, we took a road trip down to Devon, stayed at Crealy Theme Park & Resort and then headed a bit further down the country to Esplanade in Cornwall. It was an amazing trip, the ultimate in staycationing, with a spot of glamping and then a few nights in a hotel situated on one of Britain's hotspot beaches.

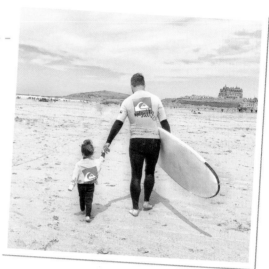

We set off on our adventure at around 5 am in an attempt to beat the traffic on our five-hour journey. Our plan is usually to get off to a good start and then, when rush hour starts to hit, we stop for some breakfast. We find it's the perfect way to skip out the really heavy traffic, and it means we're not eating super-early before we set off. Motorway stops are quite pricey but they are easier for us than stopping with a picnic. Anyway, we made really good time and, after a couple of stops, we arrived nearby just after lunch. We knew that our cabin wouldn't be ready until after 3 pm, so we drove into Torquay and visited the fabulous Torquay Dinosaur World; a small but really fun attraction that was exactly what my dino-loving kids needed after a long drive. The museum is well worth a visit. It's a little worn, but there are loads of interactive things for children to do, not to mention lots of huge dinosaur models. After we explored the museum, we went for fish and chips at the Rockfish restaurant just a little way along the street. It was so lovely to be able to sit outside and watch the comings and goings while the children played with the entertainment pack that came with the kids' meals and we had a slow lunch. You also can't beat a British seaside town for good ole fish and chips! After this, with three very tired

mini travellers, we headed back to acquaint ourselves with our home for the next three days. Crealy Theme Park & Resort is the UK's largest theme park with camping onsite too. They have the most hot tub lodges in Devon so, if you're looking for a little bit of extra luxury, it's a complete win. However, if you prefer pitching your own tent then that's an option too, and they are right on top of a fabulous children's theme park with evening entertainments for guests. There's also a restaurant where you can have a hot breakfast (recommended) and pizza. For camping guests, they have washrooms and toilets so it's a little bit more comfortable than your standard field in the middle of nowhere if you have babies or toddlers.

I'll never forget the children jumping in and out of the hot tub, despite the fact that it was raining! The theme park itself was ideal for under 10s and smaller kids as it's all very geared towards young children with lots of indoor play areas too. We self-catered for the majority of the trip, though we had to test out the pizza bar and breakfast, of course. With a Tesco only a few miles away (the weather was freezing and we had packed for sunshine so had to grab some clothes as well as food) we found it was really easy to get all the things that we needed, keep the cost of our stay to a minimum and spend it on more fun things like day trips and a few souvenirs. A few days here was the perfect pitstop for us on the way down to Cornwall, and a really fun way to experience one type of staycationing while getting to visit wonderful places like Torquay Dinosaur World and Torquay harbour.

On the final day, we enjoyed breakfast in the restaurant (chocolate chip pancakes) and then headed onwards to Newquay, Cornwall, where we stayed at the Esplanade Hotel, right on the beachfront. The Esplanade hotel offers loads of things for children to do, as well as having a few double rooms (no hiding in the bathroom while you wait for the kids to drop off to sleep here!). There are also free activities for kids to join in with, like cookie and cupcake decorating, and you can even do some paid activities like 'build a bear'! It probably goes without saying that our best memories in Cornwall centered around the beach as, whether it was rockpooling or surfing, we absolutely adored it. Even Edith, at the age of three, tried a little surfing, though admittedly her and Toby weren't keen and were out of the water fairly quickly. My favourite memories are of Reuben and Adam jumping into the experience with both feet and trying their best to ride the waves, and of finding a gorgeous little café and bar just up the road from the Esplanade Hotel, where we popped in for a coffee to warm up after some surfing.

On the final day in Cornwall, we visited the absolutely amazing Eden Project. It is a place I have always wanted to visit but it was so much more than I expected. With the most glorious gardens and

loads of play areas for the kids, it absolutely didn't disappoint.

Overall, our experiences of UK staycations have been some of the most fulfilling family holidays we have ever had. I can say with complete confidence that it's worth considering a staycation.

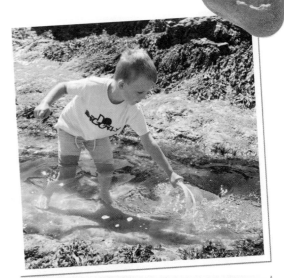

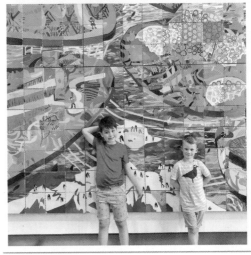

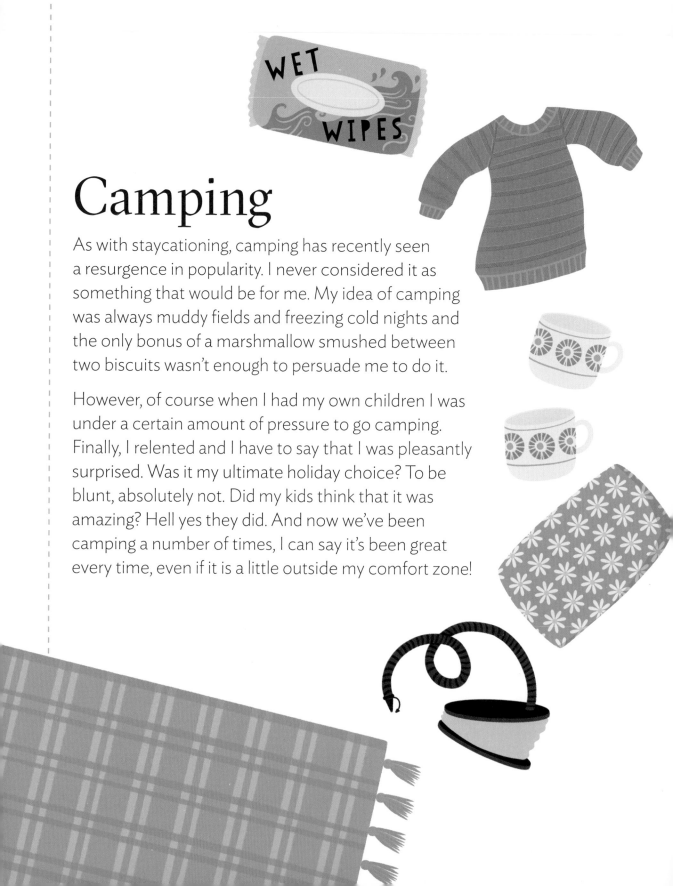

Camping

As with staycationing, camping has recently seen a resurgence in popularity. I never considered it as something that would be for me. My idea of camping was always muddy fields and freezing cold nights and the only bonus of a marshmallow smushed between two biscuits wasn't enough to persuade me to do it.

However, of course when I had my own children I was under a certain amount of pressure to go camping. Finally, I relented and I have to say that I was pleasantly surprised. Was it my ultimate holiday choice? To be blunt, absolutely not. Did my kids think that it was amazing? Hell yes they did. And now we've been camping a number of times, I can say it's been great every time, even if it is a little outside my comfort zone!

Everything you need to know about camping with kids

There are so many different ways to camp, from the traditional (and sometimes free) 'mum and dad struggle with awkward tent' vibe all the way to glamping, which is a modern way of saying 'cabin with basic amenities and not really camping at all'. It's hard to know what to do first, so my best tip would be to ease yourself in gently and begin with a campsite that provides everything, before you commit to buying all the gear yourself.

START EASY

Embers Camping sites are a brilliant way to ease yourself into camping gently. It feels like proper camping as it's in a big ole field, surrounded by nature, but the bonus is that you can choose to have a tent that is already set up for you (or set it up yourself) and there are wash facilities on site. It might mean that you have to trek across the field for a wee, but if you're nervous about a nature wee or what the hell you are meant to do if your child needs a poo (do you really bury it?!), then this is much MUCH easier. There is also a little shop across the field that sells pizza and various things like coffee and milk. Never underestimate the beauty of being able to get coffee in the morning, I say.

HAVE A BACK-UP PLAN

Expecting things to go wrong isn't necessarily a bad thing. When we first started camping with the kids, I would look up local B&Bs or work out where the local Premier Inn was so that I had a back-up plan if we were all struggling. I never actually needed it, but that route out of 'OK, Edith is shrieking endlessly. I can't cope and I'm going to bail' gave me much peace of mind.

YOU NEED AN AIR BED

I always assumed that you just lay on the floor of the tent with your sleeping bag... wrong! You need an inflatable air bed for camping, always. You can buy inflatable anything for camping now, including sofas and armchairs! Adam and I had an inflatable double, the boys had an inflatable double and Edith had a small Peppa Pig air bed, which I ordered online and that had its own blanket attached.

OVERPACK, DON'T UNDER-PACK

The first time I went camping with the kids, I was SO smug. I'd packed an ice box FULL of stuff to eat and drink, I'd packed a BBQ to cook some sausages on in the morning, cereal for the kids... gosh I was on fire, right? Hmm, not so much. I forgot cutlery, plates, cups and wet wipes (the camper's gold). We ended up having to wait until the local café opened so that we could have breakfast and the kids staved off hunger with marshmallows, biscuits and my sanity.

TAKE EXTRA BLANKETS

Even when it is really lovely weather, the temperature drops at night. We usually take our sleeping bags and a duvet or thick, heavy blanket each. Extra socks and thick PJs are also a must, in my experience.

BUY A DISPOSABLE MINI BBQ (OR A PORTABLE ONE) BUT CHECK THE CAMPSITE REGULATIONS FIRST

At the first campsite we stayed, I was surprised to find a fire pit there already (that you could buy logs for), but they didn't allow portable BBQs. If you are allowed, I think they are great but, if not, just buy logs for the fire (and don't forget the marshmallows). Don't forget to look into what the campsite offers by way of food, so you can plan ahead.

DON'T EXPECT A NORMAL BEDTIME

One of the questions I was always asked when I mentioned that I had been camping with the kids was, 'Did they go to bed OK?' And the truth is... yes... and no. They went to bed around 10 pm (three hours later than usual) but it didn't present any problems. They played in the field with the other children, enjoyed some treats and pizza around the campfire, then got into their sleeping bags and dropped off. I say, let loose and allow them to have some fun as it's not forever and they are on holiday.

EARLY RISERS MAY BE EVEN EARLIER

Before I camped, it had never occurred to me how very noisy the morning actually is. I'd always assumed it was fairly serene and quiet but, when you're outside, you realise it most certainly is not. Birds and sunlight don't make for great sleeping-in conditions.

TEST DRIVE

If you have a garden, you could always give camping a test drive and pitch a tent outside overnight! Yes, it means you have to fork out for a tent yourself, but you can find some really reasonably priced ones in supermarkets during festival season or online.

camping checklist

- [ ] Tent, if you're taking one
- [ ] Airbeds for everyone
- [ ] Sleeping bags for everyone
- [ ] Blankets
- [ ] PJs and spare clothes (extra pants)
- [ ] Chairs to sit in during the day
- [ ] BBQ/firewood
- [ ] Cooking utensils and pots and pans
- [ ] Money
- [ ] Food and snacks in a cool box
- [ ] Drinks in a cool box
- [ ] Wet wipes (or cloths if you prefer not to use wet wipes)
- [ ] First aid kit
- [ ] Emergency contact list for the campsite manager
- [ ] Battery packs and cables
- [ ] Nappies/portable potty for little ones
- [ ] Cups/plates/cutlery
- [ ] Portable speaker or radio
- [ ] Hot water bottles
- [ ] Sun cream
- [ ] Torch
- [ ] Bite/sting cream
- [ ] Any extra camping items you might want to bring like games sets, portable stoves, portable washing machines, portable showers – there are so many things, it depends on how often you camp!

Making camping extra fun

The basic elements to camping are all you need for it to be loads of fun, but there are a few little extras that can make it just a little bit... extra.

FAIRY LIGHTS

Some campsites will already have these up, but if not, I would highly recommend them. They provide a little extra light in otherwise pitch blackness, but they also instantly make things feel a bit more homely.

MARSHMALLOW CAMPING KITS

You can buy these in supermarkets, but if not, they are super-easy to put together. You need a bag of extra large marshmallows, some chocolate fondue (Nutella in a foil tray will work) and Digestive biscuits.

PORTABLE RADIO OR BLUETOOTH SPEAKERS

It makes all the difference to have some of your fave music playing (respectfully) around the campfire.

GARDEN GAMES/SPORTS STUFF

We forgot this and fortunately the campsite we went to had some bits on site, but people camping next to us took all manner of games, from badminton sets to cricket sets to human snakes and ladders boards. I wished we had thought of it. We did the next time and it was great!

GLOW IN THE DARK DUCT TAPE

No, I'm not joking. You can buy this on Amazon and I think it's perfect for drawing a little pathway to your tent, creating your own glow stick and marking places out!

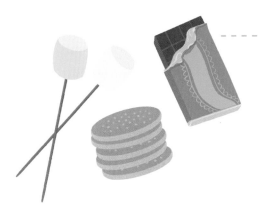

Camping vs glamping

As you can probably tell, I'm not the most enthusiastic camper. I do enjoy it with the children, mainly because they LOVE it, but I'm more of a glamper myself. Glamping can be anything from the kind of camping I've mentioned above at Embers Camping sites, where you have a tent set up and ready, amenities around you and the security of knowing that you have everything on hand, all the way to chic yurts, mini log cabins and luxury camper vans. Camping is definitely a little more rough and ready and I think, unless you are really into the wild vibe, it's not so common in the UK now. I struggle to think of many campsites that don't have, at the very least, stalls for toilets. It's also worth remembering that you can't actually just pitch a tent anywhere anymore.

notes

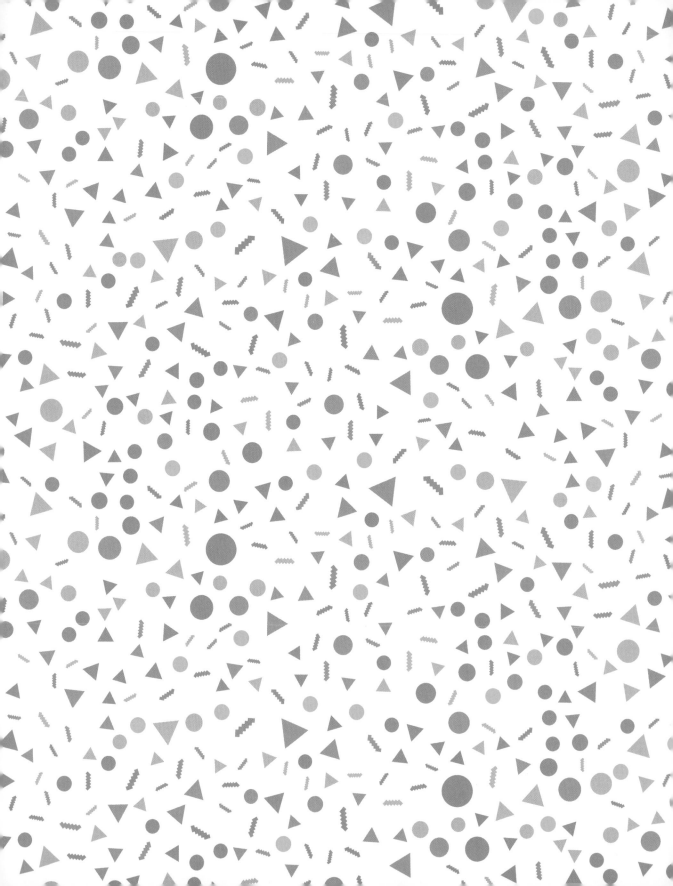

BODY & BEAUTY

When I was younger, I would spend a lot of my time obsessing about my weight. As a tween and teen, I was a large girl. Eating was my comfort and, although I was also fit and active, I was always led to believe that this was inherently wrong. **Throughout my life I have been a yo-yo crash dieter of epic proportions** and have gone from a UK size 18 to a size 8-10 and back again, more times than I care to count. And the theme that links it all? A chronic lack of self-confidence and self-esteem.

When I became a mother for the first time, I remember being bombarded with diet ads and feeling the pressure to 'lose the baby weight' almost immediately. When I started to do this, I felt great. **The compliments fueled me constantly, until I realised that my sense of self-worth was almost exclusively about my weight.** Day in and day out, the scales would determine my mood and how sexy and attractive I would feel.

When I became pregnant with Toby, I had recently lost loads of weight and was exceptionally slim. I remember feeling consumed with a fear that the pregnancy would mean that I gained it all back, as if that was more important than my overall health or the health of the baby I was carrying. I sobbed to the midwife at my 36-week weigh-in because I had gained 14lbs. How insane is that? Yet it was all I could think about. And that buttered toast that they offer you in the maternity ward after you've given birth? I didn't want to eat it because the diet started NOW. Today, looking back, it's pretty simple to see that I had a problem, but it's not an uncommon one, especially in new mums. **It's taken me years to feel happier and confident in my skin and to learn that it's more important to link my joy to the smiles on my children's faces,** the big squeezes they give me and my own achievements, rather than a number on a set of scales.

I don't want to demonise weight loss, either. I believe that, ultimately, it's your body and, if you feel that you want to change it, however that may be, then power to you. It's simply about acknowledging that, as a person, there is more to you than your weight.

We might be mothers but we're also women and, in this section of the book, I want to share with you some of the things that I do to make myself feel good, love my body and feel secure in myself. These beauty and fashion tips don't require much time at all but they help me feel like a woman, as well as a mum.

Mums, this section is dedicated to every single one of you who feels as if you're not enough, because you are.

The boob section

One (or two) of the things that change the most during pregnancy and after becoming a mum are the ole' knockers. There is no escaping it as you are not spared even if you choose not to breastfeed. It's actually the hormones in pregnancy that can convert you from perky princess to dachshund's ears in around nine months. A good bra is therefore a must and, when I worked for Mothercare, one of the things that I learnt to do was fit one properly – maternity bras and nursing bras for ladies at all stages. Most women would come in for a fitting at the very last minute and it was clear that it felt invasive and intrusive at a time when they were hormonal or feeling insecure about their changing bodies. Of course, there were also the women who didn't think twice about it and would come in, strip off and chat to you about the latest TV programme that they had been loving. It's true, bra-fitting can feel rather awkward even at the best of times, so here's a guide to bras and how to fit them so you can do it all from home. Viva la boob!

measuring yourself for a bra

1. Keeping your bra on, take a tape measure and place it under your bust. Measure your bandwidth in inches and, if it's an odd number add 5, if it's an even number, add 4.

So, a 31-inch measurement would actually put you in a 36-inch bandwidth, as would a 32-inch measurement.

2. From there, keeping your bra on, go across the nipple line to find your cup measurement. The difference between your bandwidth and your nipple line measurement gives you your cup.

So, if your bandwidth is 36 inches and your nipple line is 38 inches, that's a 2-inch difference, which makes you a B cup (see below).

0 = AA   1 = A   2 = B   3 = C   4 = D
5 = E   6 = F   7 = G   8 = H

As with everything, it's a guide and you will need to try bras on to make sure you are comfy with your size. I always think that you want to feel snug but you don't want anything squeezed or falling out.

LOOKING FOR A NURSING BRA?

Follow the same measurements and add 1–2 cups. I would always say 1 cup, unless it's a second or more pregnancy and you know you will need 2 cup increases, or your current cup is very snug.

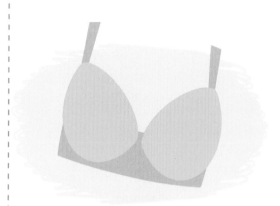

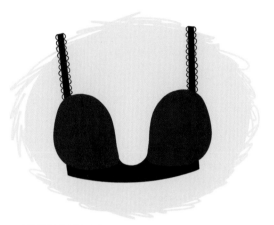

T-SHIRT/CONTOUR BRAS

The staple of the bra kingdom, these are best for full, round busts as plunges tend to dig at the sides of a larger boob. You can go for underwire or not, depending on what you feel most comfortable with. Underwire tends to be for day-to-day wear, with wireless for weekends and lounging. However, since my nursing bra days, I'm all about that comfort 24/7 and I rarely bother with wires. George at Asda offer some great, really well-priced T-shirt bras but my favourite brand is Bravissimo.

PLUNGE BRAS

These are to go with that low-cut top or dress when you want to feel a little sassy. They're all about pushing the gals together and increasing the appearance of size, so definitely not a comfy option if you are still breastfeeding as they squeeze from the side. I lived in these as a twenty-something – Victoria's Secret did the best.

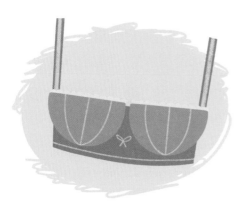

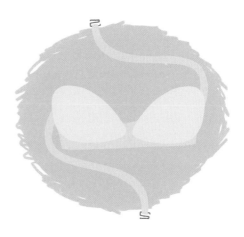

BALCONETTE BRAS

These will lift you and are ideal if you have boobs that are wider set. They are a great option for square or curved neck tops. The cup is always underwired and you want something that has a deep cup with a gentle underwire that is not as curved as a T-shirt or plunge bra. As someone with big boobs, I've never found them especially comfy or easy to wear, though Freya make a great moulded version.

CONVERTIBLE BRAS

Convertibles are the ones where the straps can go every which way or be taken off completely. Usually they will look like a T-shirt bra, but you can find plunge versions too. In my opinion, M&S is the king of this type of bra.

CHECKING YOUR BOOBS

According to Coppafeel, one in eight women will experience breast cancer in their lives, and 400 men are diagnosed every year with breast cancer. You can check your boobs anywhere, and there isn't a right or wrong way to do it – just get to know what feels normal and what doesn't. You're looking for changes in size, shape, any new thickness or lumps, any pain that isn't linked to your period, plus rashes, pimpled skin or dimples. Make sure you check under your armpits and up into your collarbone. Coppafeel suggest you check at least once a month!

Stylish in five minutes

In my experience, after you've had children, it's very easy to take a back seat in your own life. It happened to me. I would get everyone else ready, organise ALL the things they needed and then realise that I hadn't really bothered with myself at all. I would just throw on whatever was near me and go go go. I wasn't the priority anymore, and I often felt like I was 'wasting money' on clothes or nice make-up for myself, when I could replace those things with clothes for the kids or toys.

However, over the last couple of years, I've made a conscious effort to bring a little style back into my life. I've realised that it's important to remember that, just because you have children, it doesn't mean you have to lose yourself to leggings and a baggy jumper every day. You shouldn't deny yourself a little self-love as making the effort to look nice can really lift you when you're feeling flat. It doesn't even need to take long – I've worked out how to do it in five minutes. So here are a few speedy ideas on how to get stylish with timeless outfits or looks that will never let you down.

THE CLASSIC JEANS AND A TEE COMBO
The jeans and a T-shirt look is timeless and effortlessly cool. Tuck the tee into your jeans, pair with trainers or boots and a blazer and a red lip.

THE 'DONE IN ONE' DRESS
Midi dresses are so in and have been for years. They will probably never go out of style and, if they do, will simply be replaced with a new length. A dress is always a super simple way to make yourself feel a little bit chic. I team my dresses with trainers because then I can run around after my little monsters. And I like a bold, colourful dress with a nice neutral make-up look. If you're like me and worry about the ole chub rub, Snag Tights are the best for easy to wear, effortlessly simple chub rub shorts.

THE MIDI SKIRT AND TEE
As simple as the jeans and a tee look, just replace the jeans with a midi skirt – it means you don't flash your arse when you bend down to your child's level to tell them off for whatever they did this time. It's also not long enough to get dragged through puddles or on the ground. Canvas trainers look great with this one.

THE JUMPSUIT
This is another 'done in one' look. Throw on a jumpsuit, pair it with some trainers, and if you want to make it look more dressy for those work days or evenings out with friends, simply add heels. Voila!

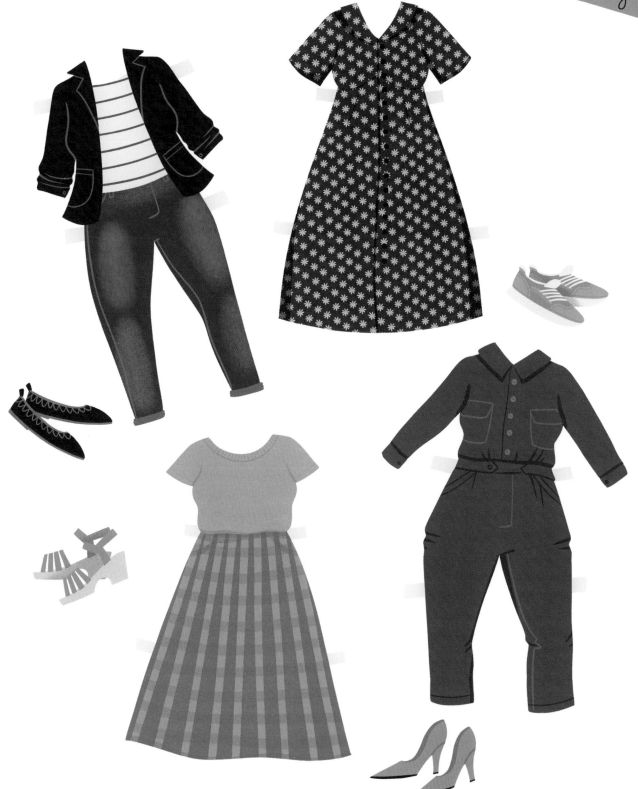

Beauty hacks

Sometimes I wake up and I look in the mirror and think HOLY SHIT, what is wrong with my face?! Who is that? I have big puffy bags under my eyes that could easily do the weekly shop, I have breakouts and I look like I've had about three hours sleep... Well, turns out I have had about three hours sleep consistently for around nine years, so that's usually why I look like shite. However, when the coronavirus pandemic hit, I started to take the time to improve my skincare routine and realised that some of the simple hacks were actually better than the all-singing all-dancing skincare products.

Homemade face masks

ESPECIALLY FUN FOR KIDS TO JOIN IN WITH TOO!

OAT MASK
FOR OILY SKIN

1 egg
½ cup (45g) oats
1 teaspoon honey
juice of 1 lemon

Mix the ingredients together, spread on the face and leave for 10–15 minutes. Alpha hydroxy acids in lemon juice remove dead skin and oil, while the oats soothe and the egg dries, which will give the skin the feeling of being pulled tighter.

COCOA YOGURT MASK
FOR SENSITIVE SKIN

2–3 tablespoons Greek yogurt
2 teaspoons cocoa powder
1–2 teaspoons honey

Mix all the ingredients together, spread on the face and leave for 10–15 minutes. Yogurt is rich in probiotics and will soothe the skin, the cocoa contains flavanol which will soothe and improve the skin's elasticity (acting as an anti-aging agent) and the honey will tighten.

BLUEBERRY MASK
FOR DULL SKIN

1 tablespoon crushed blueberries
1 tablespoon lemon juice
1 tablespoon pureed cucumber
   or cucumber water
2 tablespoons bicarbonate of soda
1–2 tablespoons water

Mix all the ingredients together, spread on the face and leave for 10–15 minutes. Blueberries are natural antioxidants, while the lemon and bicarb brighten the skin.

MOISTURISING WHEN YOUR SKIN IS STILL WET IS THE WAY FORWARD.

I usually use the not-so-natural wet jelly from Sanctuary Spa (you can find it at boots.com) but if you use any moisturiser when your skin is still wet, it will absorb more moisture. If you want a natural solution, try coconut oil or aloe vera (always test aloe vera first to ensure you aren't allergic).

BYE BYE EYE BAGS

Cold green tea bags placed under the eyes (I have used normal tea bags after my evening cuppa too...) is a really good idea for reducing eye bags without buying fancy creams. Drink lots of water and cut down on caffeine too.

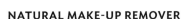

REMOVE FAKE TAN STREAKS

with a lemon juice and sugar scrub. Mix 1 cup granulated sugar with juice of ½ lemon, lemon zest and ¼ cup coconut oil. For stubborn places, add sugar to the end of a lemon and scrub neat. It stings in cuts, so be warned!

NATURAL MAKE-UP REMOVER

Coconut oil can be a natural make-up remover – it doesn't work very well on mascara (in my humble opinion) but it works incredibly well on everything else and also acts as a very effective moisturiser.

BANISH THE BREAKOUT

There are so many different ways of doing this naturally. What has always worked best for my VERY oily skin is to dab a bit of toothpaste on my spot to clear it up (it essentially dries overnight). However, this is not a good idea for dry skin; Sudocrem or any other nappy rash cream with zinc in it is gentler for your skin and really effective too.

COFFEE IS FOR MORE THAN DRINKING!

Coffee is actually hella useful – not the instant stuff but ground coffee. If you mix it with coconut oil and sugar, you have yourself an intense moisturiser and exfoliant. Mix equal quantities of sugar, coconut oil and ground coffee – I usually make a jar and use $^1/_3$ cup (about 5 tablespoons) of each.

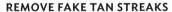

Beauty bag babes

We all have those beauty products
that we simply can't be without, right?
Here are mine:

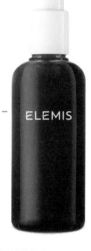

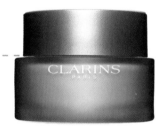

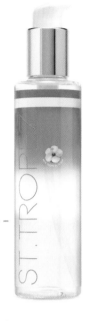

FACEWASH

I love Elemis for skincare. I'm a big
fan of their facial wash, followed
up with their cleansing balm.

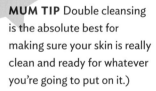

MUM TIP Double cleansing
is the absolute best for
making sure your skin is really
clean and ready for whatever
you're going to put on it.)

DAILY MOISTURISER

My absolute favourite is from
Clarins. Whilst it is aimed
specifically at dry skin, I have
combination to oily and I loved it,
it really feels dreamy on!

BODY MOISTURISER

The Sanctuary Spa wet skin
moisturiser is a huge time saver
and a way to spend 20 seconds
looking after yourself. Keep it in
the shower and when you switch
off the water, rub all over your
wet skin. Dry yourself as normal
and voila!

FAKE TAN

I was never really a fake tan user
until I discovered the St. Tropez
range. The gel is so easy to use
and it doesn't streak at all, and
their face mist is the bee's knees
for that gentle gradual glow.

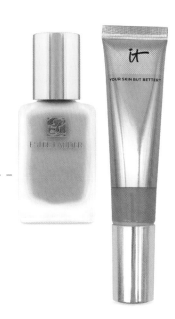

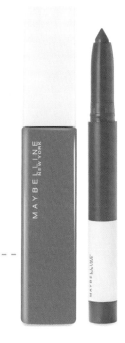

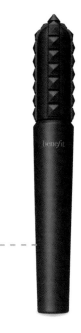

FOUNDATION

I have two in my bag that I am absolutely wild for. For the times when I want a really full cover, I wear Estée Lauder foundation. It never slides around and is still on my face when I come to the end of the day. My second foundation is the fabulous CC+ cream with SPF 50+ from IT Cosmetics. That SPF alone is wowzer, and it gives brilliant coverage and yet feels so light and airy.

LIPS

This has become a bit of a running joke amongst my friends because I almost always wear the same brand of lipstick and I'm obsessed with it. As someone who is constantly carrying around stuff for my kids, or travelling, I don't want to keep topping up and Maybelline's liquid lipstick lasts forever. I don't find it particularly drying, unlike other lip inks but, if you want something even gentler, the lip ink crayon is great too.

MASCARA AND BROWS

I use Benefit mascara and their brow styler for my brows. Both last all day and I find them really easy to use.

HIGHLIGHTER

For a natural shine and a little pick-me-up, I use one from Iconic London. A little goes a long way so it lasts forever!

How to have a bath
without the kids

STEP 1
Deploy distraction techniques. Think snacks and TV/tablets.

STEP 2
Wink to your co-parent, offer a head gesture and mouth the
word 'bath'. Ensure they don't think this is an invitation
(it's easy to confuse). NOTE: **do not** mention that you are
going for a bath, this is a guaranteed method to attract children.

STEP 3
Back out of the room. Sudden movements are discouraged.
If they ask, 'Where are you going?' simply reply, 'To clean
the toilet'. This is likely to discourage further enquires.

STEP 4
Make your way to the bathroom.

STEP 5
Run bath with your favourite bubble bath.

STEP 6
Light candles, prepare to relax.

STEP 7
Get in the bath. Enjoy for 90 seconds. That was your bath.

STEP 8
Make room for small child who has made their way
upstairs after hearing your bath running,
smelling your luxury bubble bath and fancies joining in.

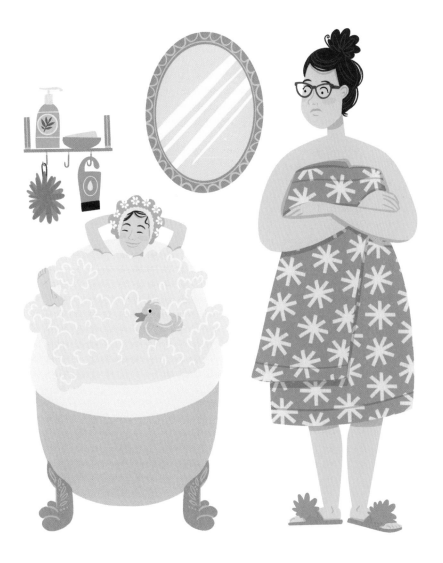

STEP 9

Add extra cold water for them and get out
so they can enjoy your bath.

STEP 10

Try again when they are over ten,
but be prepared for them to come and use the toilet or
have a chat with you until they leave home.

How to love yourself, because you deserve it

I remember being in my early twenties and wondering when, exactly, I would start to feel more confident in myself, a little less insecure about my thighs and perhaps be a bit nicer to the reflection in the mirror. After I had Reuben, I spiralled down a dark hole of self-loathing and complete lack of self-esteem. I'd gained more weight than I ever had before, I was uncomfortable in the clothes I was trying to squeeze myself into and I knew that I HAD to 'lose the baby weight' because I kept hearing the phrase over and over again. If there is one thing I have learnt over the years since then, it's that self-love is not something that you wake up and decide to have one morning. Body positivity and confidence is not something that you shrug on like a coat in the winter – it's something that is ever-changing. Some days you might feel it, but on other days you might lack any kindness towards yourself at all.

On my social media channels, I've often gone through spurts of feeling a great sense of body confidence and self-love, something I've shared and chatted to people about. My hope is to inspire them to dress how they want, appreciate their amazing selves the way they deserve to and to be, all in all, much happier inhabiting their own bodies and minds. What I don't discuss so often are the days when I feel none of those things, when I feel the insecurities creeping back in

THE POSITIVE PLANNER by Alison McDowall and Claire Finn-Prevett is great for anyone who likes to have a physical diary. Days are broken down with 'daily intentions' to be filled out and self-care reminders. Evening reflections allow you to jot down how the day went but also to acknowledge positive things from the day, no matter how small. It was designed by two women who both suffered with mental health problems and felt the need to create something to help them to focus on the good.

when I look at an old photo and silently think 'I wish I was as thin as I was then'. The logical part of me remembers how I was never satisfied with my body, was always critical, forever hungry, and basically had an eating disorder that I couldn't talk about to anyone.

Here's the thing: body confidence and self-love aren't static. On some days, you won't have to work very hard to be kind to yourself, and on other days it will be an uphill battle in a blizzard. However, no matter how hard it is, you deserve your own kindness.

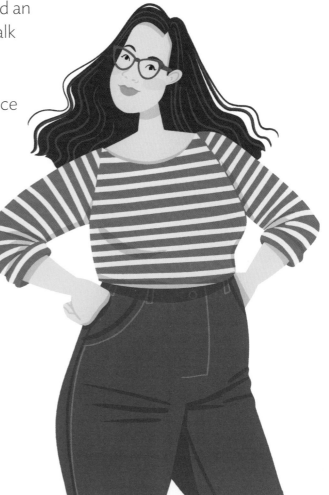

a few of the things I do to be kinder to myself:

Buy clothes that fit you and you like, not what you think you should be allowed to wear.

I used to think that, if I only kept clothes that didn't really fit me or if I bought them a little too small, then they would force me to lose weight. Not only did this not really work for me, but it meant that I spent a significant amount of my time feeling uncomfortable and unhappy. Don't do it.

Learn to say NO

It's actually a really important thing to learn to say, 'No'. No to things that make you unhappy, no to requests that stretch you to the point of breaking. And it's not just no to the negative situations, but no to friends and family coming over if you just need some quiet time to yourself. You can always say no.

Ditch 'mum guilt' – it's a social construct

Have you ever noticed that there is no such thing as 'dad guilt'? Well, that is because mum guilt is a social construct and it is utter rubbish. You deserve better than to make yourself feel guilty for going back to work, or for being a little bit late to collect your kids from school. You are enough, and you are doing enough.

Focus on your achievements each day, no matter how small.

It doesn't matter how great or small these achievements are, I'm willing to bet that there will be plenty. It might be something huge that you have done at work, like getting a promotion or securing flexible working, or simply that you managed to get the laundry on and your kids had a clean set of PE shorts. It's not about the size of the achievement, it's about recognising that on each day there are things that you do that make a difference. Make a mental note every time you tick something off your to-do list or achieve an unexpected win. Make it your last thought before you go to sleep: I did XYZ today and that was great.

Exercise because you want to and enjoy it, not for an end goal of weight loss

Exercise for you, not for weight loss. Do it if you enjoy it, so that you get that endorphin kick.

Find five minutes a day for you

It doesn't have to be anything wild, just five minutes to wash your face, cleanse and apply some moisturiser. Maybe for you it's five minutes to read a book or five minutes to have a hot drink. I'm a firm believer that we can always 'find five'.

Mum's mantras

A mantra is essentially a word or phrase that you repeat to yourself over and over and that helps centre the mind. It originated in Buddhism and Hinduism and was a sequence of words or sounds in Sanskrit that were believed to have a mystical or magical power. I used to think that it was a bit of a waste of time, but the truth is, if you say something to yourself often enough, you start to believe it and a carefully chosen mantra can carry you through your day.

I am the expert in my own child. I trust my parental instincts.

Plenty of times I've fallen victim to unsolicited advice, especially on social media when I became very involved in Facebook groups – it made me feel like I was doing everything wrong on more than one occasion. You aren't. You are the expert in your own child, and if you feel that they aren't being supported enough at school, or perhaps in a medical capacity, it's up to you to follow your instinct and say 'I need you to listen to me and do more/differently/better'. You're their advocate, you're the expert in your child.

I can do anything, not everything.

I often guilt trip myself because I feel I haven't done enough, but the truth is that I can do anything I set my mind to but I cannot do everything. It simply isn't possible and something has to give. It is OK to ask for help, regardless of whether that help is telling a family member you need them to do more or asking a medical professional for help if you're feeling low and not yourself.

I am a good mum having a bad day.

When you are having a shitty day, it is incredibly easy to fall into the trap of thinking that you are a bad mum. You aren't. You're a great mum having a bad day and that is completely normal.

I'm doing my best and that is enough.

You are enough. Remind yourself of this frequently, especially in those moments when you feel that mum guilt is creeping in. Your best is enough, even when it doesn't feel like it.

Everything is a phase, nothing lasts forever.

Whether it's the baby phase, or a trying phase in your child's development or just a really shitty time at work, this will always be true – everything is a phase and will pass at some point. I find this really useful to repeat to myself when I'm having a bad day and I feel the kids are driving me to the point of tears.

Today doesn't have to be perfect to be wonderful.

Now, I don't know about you, but I am a bit of a planner. There have been countless times when I have planned a family day out and put so much effort into everything that I have *almost* completely ruined the day by becoming so fixated on it being exactly how I have created it in my head. When you have kids – in fact even without them – things rarely go 100 per cent to plan. Perfection isn't all it's cracked up to be, your days do not need to be perfect in order to be wonderful.

notes

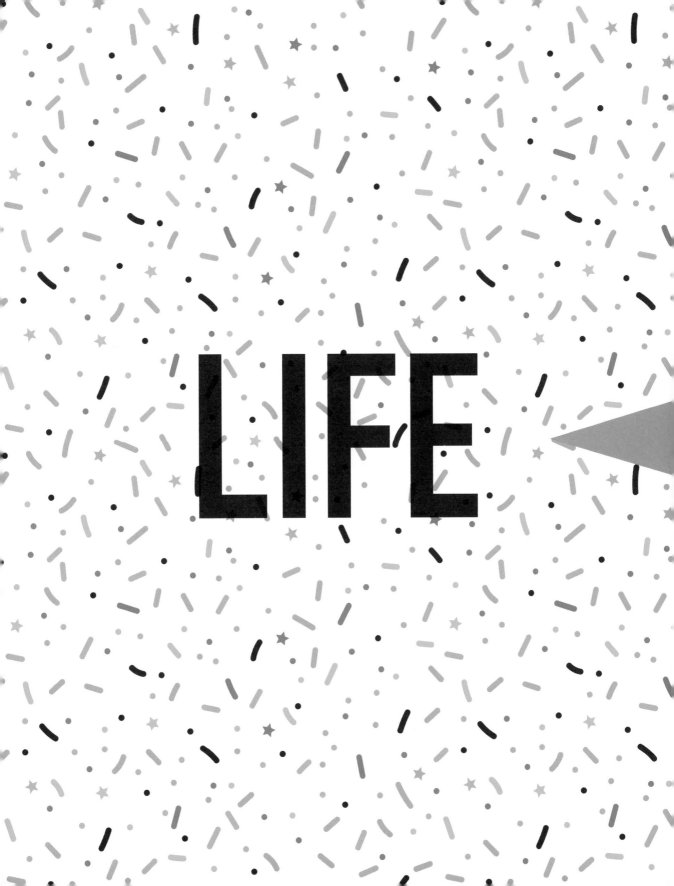

One of the truest clichés of motherhood is that 'everything changes when you have children'. **Your life is suddenly flipped 180 degrees and you view everything through an entirely new lens.** Your priorities become totally different overnight as this new little human takes centre stage. Your relationships and achievements from before matter a little less as nothing feels as important or as all-consuming as being a mother.

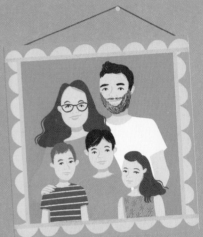

Yes, motherhood IS all-consuming. In those first few months, everything is about this new little being in your life, the little being you are responsible for keeping alive. They are your first consideration, before you do anything. You plan every move around their feeding schedules, their nap times, their nappy changes. **Going to the supermarket becomes a military operation that requires supplies, pit stops and willpower.** Friends and family coming over are suddenly a less welcome thought and more of a 'Hmm, will they disturb the baby?' or 'Is your mum going to spend the whole time telling me how I should be doing things again?'

In my own experience, I felt this to varying degrees with each child and, after my first, there were added layers of guilt each time because a small part of me felt the need to protect my smallest addition from their sibling(s). It felt like a primal urge to push the older ones away, as if they were something dangerous, despite also desperately wanting to encourage a sibling bond. When you think about it, it is completely normal because toddlers and young children are potentially dangerous to newborn babies if they aren't supervised... but try telling that to me as I sobbed to Adam because I felt like I was a terrible mother for the way my feelings had changed towards the boys when Edith first arrived.

However much you swear that it won't happen to you, your own identity does start to fade over the first few months of motherhood. I think it happens to both parents to a certain degree, but especially to mothers. After the first couple of weeks when you're in a blissful bubble of newness together, everyone and often your partner too, starts to go back to normality and you get left behind. **It can be a really odd and isolating feeling being 'someone's mum'** and wanting to feel close and attractive to your partner and to go for a coffee with friends but also feeling exhausted and lonely and afraid of your colicky baby shrieking in the café while everyone stares.

As with everything in motherhood, this feeling passes, but it takes time and I think there is a misconception that, one day, things go back to pre-child normal, which I don't agree with at all. You're always 'someone's mum', from the moment you get pregnant and, while there are moments when you reclaim the pre-child feelings – returning to work post-maternity leave or going out without the kids as a group of adults – there will always be a part of you that's blocked off and reserved for motherhood. However, I like to think of this as an addition to your character, not a detraction.

Me, you and a child too

The relationship that I feel changed the most when I had children was my relationship with my husband, but not at all in the negative way that is so often portrayed in the media. I feel like our children have brought us closer together in so many ways and I never find him more attractive than when I see him throwing our daughter into the air or snuggling one of our babies in his arms. To see his love is to fall in love with him over and over again. There is a joy in knowing that these children are ours; little extensions of ourselves who we made together because we love one another.

In 2019, a study by Channel Mum and The Baby Show showed that over a fifth of couples separate during the first year of their baby's life. The most common reasons cited were lack of sex, lack of communication and constant arguments.

Having children was definitely the making of us as a couple and made us grow up. I truly believe that. In the early days, with babies, we were of course more tired and often had a short fuse with one another. Sometimes, we'd barely bother to communicate at all and of course this widened the gap between us, allowed discontent to grow and led to the darkest dips in our marriage to date. And now that the kids are older, we still can't always find the time to talk, as we're constantly interrupted by little voices. For a long time we led very different lives, and it felt like we were passing ships in the night, certainly not lovers and not even really friends anymore. We were too tired to do anything; too tired to file for divorce and deal with the complications it would cause, and too tired to work out how to bring back the spark.

At that time, Adam worked in hospitality, which meant that he worked long hours and needed to catch up sleep at the weekend. This then made me feel resentful and I'd be enraged when he wanted to go off to football and chill out with friends when he had seen so little of us. At times, it felt like he was closer to a lot of his work colleagues than to us and, I think, if he were honest, he probably felt he was too. All we did was bicker. I was on maternity leave or working part-time as a retail assistant (while also pregnant with baby number two) and I felt lonely and unwanted. It took work to keep us going, a lot of persistence and a desire to make it, however hard it became. The main takeaway that I have when it comes to my relationship and having children is that it needs to be nurtured and it takes effort and time – from both sides.

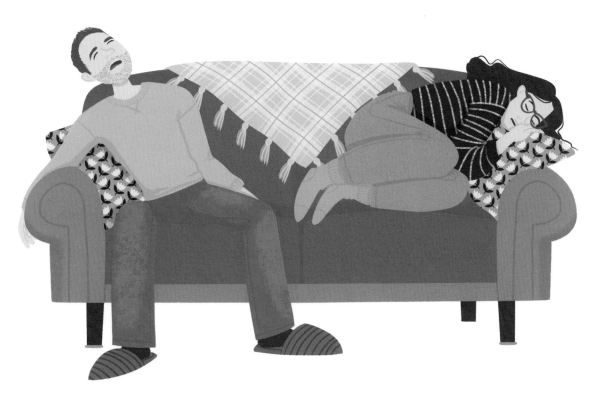

Date your partner (without a babysitter)

Making time for one another is one of the hardest things, and with that acknowledgement comes a heap of guilt because it shouldn't be taxing to spend time with your partner. However, sometimes it just is. When you're knackered, your boobs are killing you and there has just been no end to the day, the last thing you might want to do is spend 'quality time' with someone. On top of the emotional/physical reasons for not bothering to date one another, there are the logistical reasons too – who is going to babysit while you two rekindle your fire?

Here are a few really simple ideas for date nights with your partner that don't require any babysitter.

MEAL FOR TWO AT THE DINING TABLE

Will it be completely uninterrupted? Probably not, but just making an effort to sit together after the little ones have gone to bed without the interruption of the TV or your phones can make a world of difference. Talking to one another about your days, or funny things you have seen online or, well, anything, can help you to remember each other as more than mum and dad. M & S Meals for 2 are great value and feel like something a little bit special, or you can go for something even simpler, like a takeaway.

PLAY A BOARD GAME

Yep, I know, it might sound utterly wild when you're both tired and can't be arsed to do anything, but we have spent many an evening giggling away to Scrabble or something similar – just avoid Monopoly and Game of Life and you'll be fine...

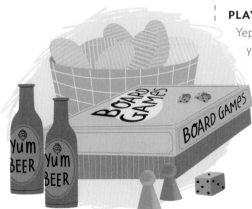

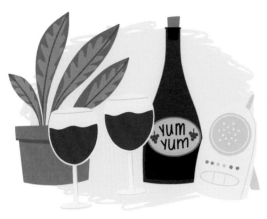

GARDEN DATE

A little time outside on a picnic blanket with a glass of something refreshing, relaxing in the sunshine with the baby monitor at your side can do you the world of good. It *almost* feels like you're somewhere else. When we took the boys on holiday for the first time, we spent every evening together on the balcony and we have both said that those were some of our favourite moments from the holiday, just getting to spend some time chatting in the warm air with a drink. In winter, there is nothing nicer than lying in a hammock or on loungers in the cool, dry air under a tonne of blankets (with maybe a hot water bottle) as you look up at the stars. It sounds corny but it's just something different from the constant TV and sofa.

HOME CINEMA

Curl up together and watch a movie. This is what we do when we are feeling a bit disconnected. We make some nachos (our fave), grab some chocolate or sweets and sit on the sofa together, phones away, to just enjoy some quiet time together.

HAVE DINNER IN BED WITH A MOVIE

Will you fall asleep? Probably, but there is still something really awesome about having a super-early night after the kids have gone to bed and tucking into pizza together as you watch a movie.

HAVE A GAMING NIGHT

I used to LOVE Crash Bandicoot as a teen, so why not enjoy a blast from the past and have a gaming night together. Go for something you will both enjoy (there's absolutely no point me playing Fifa against Adam because I will lose, he will get annoyed when it's like playing a four year old and I will hate every second), order pizza and drink a beer or whatever. Just go with it.

BOOK CLUB FOR TWO

Now this one would never work for us as Adam isn't really much of a fiction reader, but we could easily apply the same thing to a movie plot. With a book club for two, read the same book and, once a week, review your book together over some wine and cheese. It's simple, it's low cost and it's just a chance to chat.

GET INTIMATE

Nope, I'm not talking about the dance with no pants, I'm talking about having a bubble bath together, massaging each other, cuddling in bed together and talking about all your hopes and dreams. Intimacy is often thought of as sex, but you can have sex with anyone, it's sharing your everything and being open with your partner that makes them your partner.

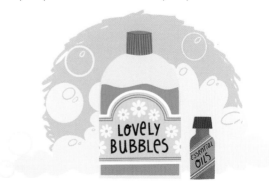

Date your partner (babysitter edition)

I genuinely think that one of the hardest things is finding a babysitter who you are both happy with. Grandparents aren't always an option, and while friends and family members say they are willing to help, it doesn't always feel right to ask. It is a bit of a minefield to be honest. Bubble App is excellent at giving you access to various qualified/checked babysitters within your area and it even allows you to see if you know anyone who has used their services, but it depends on your comfort level. Regardless, the first step for me in ensuring that your date night goes smoothly is making sure that you are both 100 per cent happy with who is looking after your child. A great alternative, if you don't have access to a babysitter and you're not comfortable hiring someone, is to book a day off work together when your little one is at a nursery or school.

MEAL FOR TWO

Going out to eat is my absolute favourite thing in the world. It doesn't have to be anywhere fancy and I often find the simplest places are the best. A drink or two before or after if time allows is always a bonus.

CINEMA

There's nothing like a traditional cinema trip. We like to combine it with a meal before or after, even if it's nothing fancy! I also think it's worth noting that, just because you're on a date, doesn't mean you have to see the exact same movie. If you have really different tastes, go together, watch different films and then go for coffee or a drink to discuss afterwards.

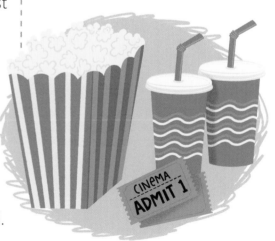

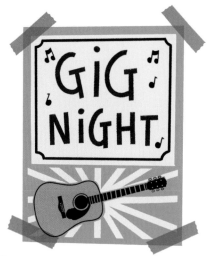

GO TO A GIG

If gigs are your thing then try going together, instead of with friends!

COMEDY SHOW

We used to do this all the time and it was always SUCH a good time. We're not too far from Hull and Leeds so we normally grab tickets and then go for an early meal together before the show. I always think it's better if it's a comedian you both enjoy, otherwise one of you feels a bit awkward if you don't find it funny.

GO APE

Go Ape, ZipWorld and so many others offer experiences for the more adventurous that you just can't do with small children in tow. In fact, finding something like this that is far removed from the child-friendly sphere is a great way to remind yourselves that you're more than parents to one another.

PICNICS IN THE PARK

Usually a fairly inexpensive date and, if you want to make it a little different, order a pizza and collect it to eat in the park together.

ESCAPE ROOM

Both Adam and I work flexibly now, so we are able to plan day dates when we have a gap in our schedules while the kids are at school. One of my favourite dates in recent memory was going to an escape room. I fully expected to hate it but actually it ended with me suggesting we book another! I didn't think an escape room would be my bag, the concept is that you are 'locked' in a room, and you solve clues using only what is in the room to make your great escape (though you aren't actually locked in the room for safety reasons and you can forfeit at any time). It was such fun and we actually worked together really well, without getting on each other's nerves or bickering – a miracle to be frank.

SPA DAY

This is something I've always wanted to do with Adam but he just isn't that keen. If it's your bag, it's well worth finding a deal for an overnight stay as the treatments are often included and it works out roughly the same price as a single spa day with a couple of treatments.

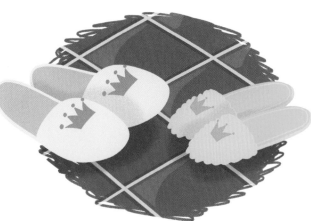

Getting back in the saddle

Sex is almost always what landed you the job of being parents so, for the majority of couples, it's a pretty huge part of a relationship. However, after you have had a baby and you've done the initial recovery period, it can feel really weird thinking about bumping uglies again. Maybe you had a difficult delivery and the thought of your partner coming within 10 feet of your newly repaired vagina makes you feel like throwing up hands. Maybe you're desperate to get back in the sack but your partner is hitting the breaks because he's worried about hurting you, or you simply aren't sure how to talk about it.

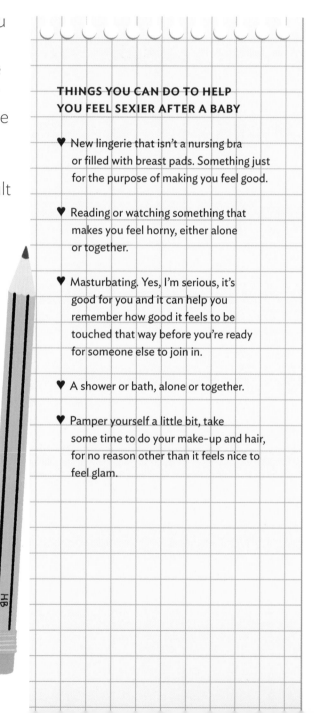

THINGS YOU CAN DO TO HELP YOU FEEL SEXIER AFTER A BABY

♥ New lingerie that isn't a nursing bra or filled with breast pads. Something just for the purpose of making you feel good.

♥ Reading or watching something that makes you feel horny, either alone or together.

♥ Masturbating. Yes, I'm serious, it's good for you and it can help you remember how good it feels to be touched that way before you're ready for someone else to join in.

♥ A shower or bath, alone or together.

♥ Pamper yourself a little bit, take some time to do your make-up and hair, for no reason other than it feels nice to feel glam.

Whatever you are feeling, it's normal. There are so many things discussed in the antenatal classes, so many helpful diagrams to prep you for the imminent birth of your little bundle, but very little to prepare you for life afterwards. And even if it was a subject that was discussed, would it go anywhere? It never ceases to amaze me that we can talk openly about the first post-baby poo, but talking about sex is met with gawfs and 'I wouldn't worry about that for a while'.

After having our children, we waited different lengths of time to get back to the dance with no pants, so the one thing that I think is key is communication. Not ready? Tell your partner. Ready, but anxious? Tell your partner. Ready and rampant? TELL. YOUR. PARTNER. It sounds like common sense and you would think that talking to the person you have a child with about sex would be really easy, but I remember first-hand the fear of rejection. What if he didn't want to because I was all leaky boobs and saggy belly? What if he didn't find me attractive anymore? What if my vagina has become the horrifying foretold bucket? I also remember, especially after Edith, that I'd suddenly be wracked with insecurity and anxiety during the main event, which did nothing to help the mood. Eventually, I communicated this to Adam and was met with nothing but love, overwhelming reassurances and tenderness. Remember, your partner isn't a mind reader, but they are your partner and, if they care about you the way they should, then your enjoyment and happiness is as crucial to them as theirs is to you.

Communication, above all, is key.

So, what if you're not ready or in the mood but you really want to be? Again, in my experience this is normal. As a new mother, you're being touched and needed so relentlessly, 24/7, that it's understandable if a part of you (your libido) has, like an overworked engine, sputtered to a halt and can't respond to more touching and more needing. If you're wanting to get back into the swing of things but you don't feel sexy or in the mood, I've found that doing something together that doesn't necessarily have the expectation of sex, but just allows you feel adult again can be really useful, and sometimes it is just bloody well going for it can remind you how much you used to enjoy it.

As with everything after a baby, if you're really not feeling like yourself and think you are struggling more than you should be, talk to a medical professional – advocate for yourself and refuse to be dismissed. You have a right to enjoy sex and your own body.

Friendship

One of the things that I found really hard to cope with when I had children was the way friendships changed. Friends who don't have children, or who have older children and a little more freedom, know that you will struggle to make it to events and, slowly but surely, they stop asking you. You start to feel like you're being left out or just plain forgotten. Work colleagues chat to each other about things that you missed while you were on maternity leave and other mum friends are in the same boat as you, with little time for hanging out. You might think you're starting to make a whole new set of friends from baby groups, all with *exactly* the same trials and tribulations as you and then, all of a sudden, the end of maternity leave looms and you hardly see one another at all.

There are so many people who have these experiences, and as an adult it can be a hard pill to swallow. But regardless of what you might think, you aren't alone.

Sorry, I can't make it!

If I had a penny for every time I had to cancel a plan because something came up with one of my little ones, I would be a rich woman. And I would be even richer if I were honest and fessed up to the number of times I cancelled plans because I was simply too tired and overwhelmed to be around other people. Friendship is a two-way street and, if you are the cancel queen, then it's no wonder that some friendships start to drift. Motherhood is so all-consuming that often it can be hard to see that it's not them stepping away from you, but in fact you withdrawing.

Why are you cancelling?

Is it something unavoidable, like your child being unwell? If that is the case, then there is little you can do. It's not always something that you can't fix though – maybe it's a case of being so exhausted that you double-booked by mistake, in which case be honest and ask your friends if you can reschedule. Sometimes, turning up late really is better than never. There have been times when I've cancelled plans because I just wanted to go to bed and, while that's understandable, occasionally I think I've distanced myself from friends under the guise of being too tired when I would actually have enjoyed a few hours of adult company, had I pushed myself to go.

A FEW SUGGESTIONS IF YOU'RE FEELING ON THE BRINK OF A CANCELLATION:

★ Take your little one with you, if something has come up. This isn't always the worst thing in the world. I have friends who are single parents and frequently have no other option but to bring their little ones to our girls' nights.

★ Go, even if you have decided you don't want to, because sometimes we all need a kick up the arse to remember that we aren't just here to be parents. Go out for drinks or meals and leave earlier if need be, but go.

★ Keep a diary, whether it is physical or digital, write everything down and get into the habit of checking it in the mornings. You'll be less likely to double-book yourself.

★ Talk to your friends. Maybe you've not long had a baby and you don't feel comfortable going out, maybe you are struggling with childcare - girls' nights in can be just as fun. If these are real friends, talk to them and be honest.

★ Text check-ins are a godsend. I think if there is one thing that Coronavirus Lockdown taught us, it's that you don't have to physically see one another to be there for each other. I had an almost weekly check-in with one of my closest friends, just to see how she was and what she was up to.

The invite must have been lost in the post

Sometimes it's nothing to do with you, your friendships drift apart, and you notice your friends getting together and you've not been invited. It can be one of the hardest parts of motherhood – watching old friends, who you used to see most weekends, getting together without you, or even work colleagues forgetting to invite you to the work do because you're not really at work at the moment.

It doesn't always matter how adaptable you try to be. If your friendship group has consisted of people who don't have children, suddenly adapting to one is a huge task. When the initial 'wahhh how cute, you've got a baby!' wears off, so does the excitement at having that baby coming as your plus one. When you have had to turn down the umpteenth invite to a booze-fuelled day sesh, you will sometimes find that people stop inviting you altogether. It's just the way the cookie crumbles – life is not a sitcom where everyone is besties forever.

Girls' night in

Girls' night in is one of my absolute fave things to do. It started with Ann Summers parties in the early noughties and has evolved into something a little bit more sophisticated... and by that I mean there are fewer vibrators but still the same volume of snacks and hilarious booze-fuelled giggles. Having your friends over for a few drinks really feels like the perfect mum solution to friendship for me. You can stay in your comfies, everyone brings their own booze and you can even chip in together for a takeaway or just bring some nibbles.

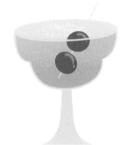

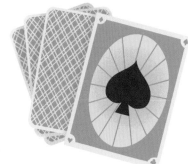

GIN OR COCKTAIL NIGHT

A simple gin or cocktail night (maybe mocktail for the designated drivers) with some different chips 'n' dips is always a winner. There is nothing quite like a catch up with a few drinks and I would say this is the staple of any friendship

HOME SPA

Not just for the teens and tweens. We seem to think that, once we get to a certain age, we can no longer have a spa get-together with friends unless it's in swanky spa setting, but actually that's not true. If everyone brings along a face mask and some nail polish, it can be a really simple pampering night that costs very little. Alternatively, you can now hire spa professionals who come to your home and run a spa session for you.

GAMES NIGHT

Who said gaming was just for guys? If you are a gamer and your friends are too, go for it. If computer gaming isn't your bag, what about something like a board games and nibbles with drinks. Think outside the box – it never hurts and you can always default to just drinks and chatter.

TV FINALE GET TOGETHER

Order some pizzas or buy some from the supermarket and have friends over to watch the end of a TV series you have all been watching. It could be the cheesiest reality TV series or a movie you've all been waiting for, but having everyone together can be a really lovely chilled night.

CAKE AND A CUPPA

Not everything has to revolve around booze (I mean, it's certainly helpful!) so try a cake and cuppa night. Just have a chat and put the world to rights.

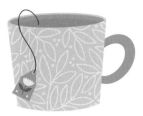

Mum's first night out

I'll never forget the first time I went out with the girls after having Reuben. I ended up absolutely RUINED. Completely. I went from being able to having a glass of wine or two on a weekday after work and feeling nothing to not being able to take a sniff of wine without feeling giddy! So, here are a few things you should know about that first night out...

1. I think it's less the booze and more the sense of freedom, of having a certain amount of time where you're not in demand, where someone doesn't need to grab your boob or throw up on you.

2. You will feel irrationally excited about the fact that your handbag doesn't need to carry ALL the things like nappies and wipes and bottles and changes of clothes. It will be small, gloriously small and of course you will need to point out this fact to at least one person – 'look how small it is!'

3. You will probably tell yourself that you should cancel at least once or twice – DON'T, you deserve a break from time to time.

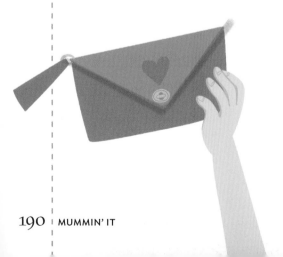

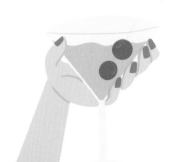

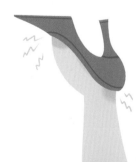

4. It's all fun and games until you feel a wet patch on your boobs, so make sure your bag is big enough for breast pads!

5. You're going to talk about your baby. A LOT! Probably to anyone who will listen, including strangers.

6. There will be a ridiculous level of excitement at being out with loud music and friends. You'll feel like a nineteen year old again... until around 11 pm/12 am when you will turn back into a pumpkin and 100 per cent need your bed. Wild.

7. You will need to check in on the baby repeatedly. Possibly every 30–40 minutes. Make sure your phone is charged.

8. In the same way that your body has forgotten how to handle even a whiff of booze, your feet have shunned heels.

9. That first hangover will be horrific. How did they get worse because you had a baby?!

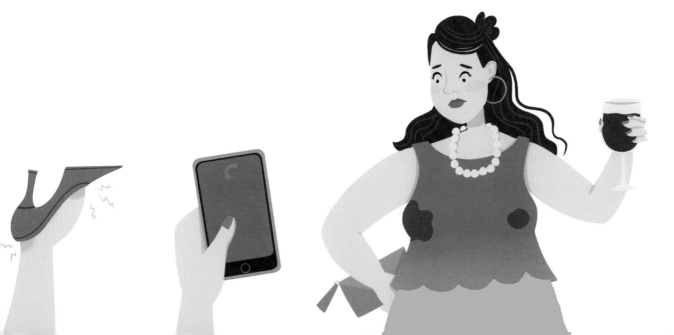

Work

Ahh, that work/life balance. If you type 'work/life balance' into Google, you will find a BAJILLION hits, all telling you about this balance and how to achieve it. It sounds like things that you can put into practice, but in reality, I'm not a fan.

I guess the easiest way to think about work/life balance is as a set of scales – if you put a little bit more into your work sometimes (which is exactly what I'm doing now FYI, now the kids have gone to bed with a rapid story and a threat to not leave their rooms) then the work side goes up, but your life side goes down a little. It's not to say that you can't have ANY balance, but when you read about the fabled 'work/life balance', it makes it sound like you are going to crack the balance and be done. I'm here to tell you, you're not. The work/life balance that we have been told about doesn't work, because it's not a quick fix or a one-off thing that you make exist. You will constantly have to juggle, or refigure things as life changes or chucks you a curve ball, and that isn't because you failed to balance your work or your life and marry them together like a happy little couple. It's always a conundrum.

Ultimately, when you find yourself in a situation where your work or your life aren't playing nice, you have to remember that it is not forever. Speak to people and ask for help and, if you can't do that, then work out how to re-jiggle the balance of those scales. Above all, remember that the person at the centre of the scales is YOU. You have the power to tip them back into place, even if it feels like you don't and you can't let one or the other completely override your wants and needs.

Work

Time/day obligation
Working with a team
Clients/customers
Requesting time off
Admin
Staying late/early
Sense of self-achievement
Management/managing

Life

Kids
School/Nursery life
Extended family
Friends
Partner
'Me time'
Food shopping/cooking
Life admin e.g. bills

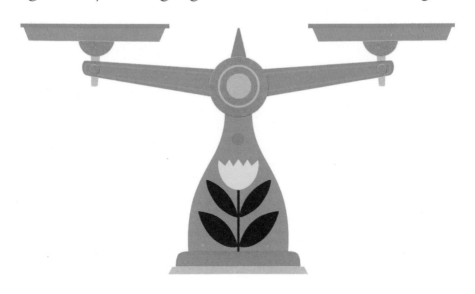

Working mum guilt word search

As I've been writing this book, I've been thinking a lot about working mum guilt. I started writing at the beginning of the pandemic, which meant a lot of 'yes, darling, if you could just go and do something with your toys Mummy will be along soon, I just need to finish this.' This would then be followed with 'Edith, I DID say I was coming, go ask Daddy,' and eventually 'WILL YOU JUST LET ME FINISH THIS PAGE AND I WILL GET YOU A *whispers swear word* SNACK!!!!!!'

My solution to working mum guilt, or any mum guilt, is obvious – don't have kids. Yes, that's right, and I realise I'm probably telling you this a touch too late if you have made it this far through the book or you're looking to find advice on precisely this subject. But, erm, it's all I've got. What is it with us mums and our guilt about everything? Can we blame the patriarchal society that tells us we should 'have it all', thus dooming us to fail because of course you can't please everyone 24/7? However, regardless of what causes it, we need to deal with it as, the more mothers I speak to, the more I realise it's not just me. We all seem to be burdened with guilt, especially around working and parenting.

I've tried many things in an attempt to offload the guilt. I tell the children 'Mummy is working and this is really important because I want to show you that you can be anything if you work hard and put your mind to it!' Or I lock away my phone on a weekend to spend unadulterated time with my children, who invariably wonder what I'm doing staring at them so intently and trying to engage them in conversations. After the first hour or so and I get 'go way Mama'.

Ultimately, then, the solution is to time jump, to not have kids and lock yourself in a nunnery, because beyond that I think motherhood (and, in particular, modern working motherhood) will always come with some kind of guilt factor. And when it all gets a bit much, when horrendous traffic means I'm the last parent at the school gates and the teacher who's had to wait with my children is scowling at me, I try to remind myself of the wonderful life I'm working at being able to give my kids, and how I love them so fiercely and unconditionally and I AM enough. I'm doing my best and that's all I've got.

find the words in bold

You are committing **SELF-SABOTAGE** – you are doing an amazing job, even if you think you aren't.

Let go of your **DOUBT**. You are a good mum.

You are not a **BAD MUM** at all.

You might feel **FRUSTRATED**, but you can't be in two places at once.

You might feel you have **NO TIME** to do all the things you want. Let something go, it won't be the end of the world.

I promise you, you're not **FAILING**.

You might feel you're **MISSING OUT** sometimes. You're not alone. Everyone feels that way, even if it's not true.

This is not **IMPOSSIBLE**. You are doing it.

TRUST yourself.

Ignore **CRITICISM** – other people's opinions don't matter.

S	D	O	U	B	T	R	Y	A	K	B	E	Z	W
C	E	H	X	I	E	R	C	S	G	N	I	G	U
V	N	L	T	P	H	E	S	C	U	O	M	I	S
U	X	O	F	R	U	S	T	R	A	T	E	D	Y
C	J	C	A	S	P	T	E	Q	T	I	O	R	H
R	B	X	I	E	A	F	G	K	C	M	C	D	R
I	N	Y	L	Q	W	B	S	H	Y	E	F	L	T
T	Z	V	I	A	E	A	O	X	V	W	N	V	U
I	C	S	N	M	U	D	A	T	R	U	S	T	Y
C	O	A	G	H	J	M	T	S	A	O	N	E	M
I	P	M	K	M	C	U	D	U	F	G	C	S	T
S	G	B	C	L	I	M	S	M	P	O	E	D	I
M	I	S	S	I	N	G	O	U	T	H	G	C	N
S	U	I	M	P	O	S	S	I	B	L	F		F

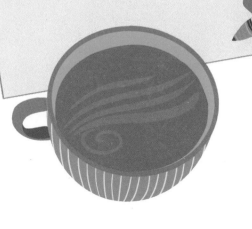

Ways to reduce stress

Even if you are the most laid-back person in the world, every so often stress will come along and thoroughly wipe the floor with you. I live my life on a more-or-less permanent stress high. Adam frequently tells me that I won't make it past 40 if I can't learn to chill out. Whether that is because I drive myself to an early heart attack or because he's silently plotting my doom, I've never worked out.

Stress can stop us from wanting to eat or make us eat more, it can make us exhausted but unable to get rest. It affects everyone differently, so it's hard to suggest a one-size-fits-all fix. It's there lurking in our lives somewhere and, no doubt, bad habits have been developing over years, in our bid to keep the ole show on the road. Then, suddenly, BOOM, along comes a baby or the terrible twos, or SATS exams, and you encounter stress like you have never known it before.

HOWEVER, THERE ARE THINGS THAT YOU CAN DO TO COMBAT IT, AND HERE'S HOW.

1. Get out in the fresh air and move your body. There is something about being surrounded by nature and inhaling fresh air that soothes the soul. I don't know if that is because we're all bound to nature or some other philosophical nonsense, but it works. Life feels brighter and we can breathe easier after a walk or jog (I will never be stressed enough to jog, OK?), and even if that isn't an option, being outside, moving in any way you are able, will still help. I have always said 'I've got so much on, I can't possibly fit in a walk' but you can, you always can.

2. Avoid hitting the bottle. I've fallen into the mum's in-joke of gin-o'clock or mummy's special grape juice, but in reality, alcohol does bugger all to solve your problems and is only likely to increase your stress levels. Drinking more water can be a really good way to keep your body hydrated and you will feel less foggy.

3. Did you know that playing something as simple as solitaire on your phone or doing sudoku puzzles can help with stress? It can. If you are feeling totally overwhelmed, try taking five minutes to play a little game, it's almost like it disconnects and then reconnects the brain.

4. Ditch the negative words. Ever had a complete crisis and thought 'I can't do this. I can't do this'? Of course you have, you're human. And if you have had a baby and never once thought 'FUCKKKKK I CAN'T DO THISSSS' then please do write to me and tell me how. All joking apart, negative words breed negative emotions, so try to avoid them.

5. Talk about it. The old saying, 'a problem shared is a problem halved' is true to an extent. It might not be halved, it might not be changed at all, but it can feel like a really good release to be able to say 'hey, this is what is happening, I feel this way about it. Can you just listen?' Talk to your partner, talk to your friends or family or even random strangers – just get it out. And If you really feel you can't talk to anyone about your stress, then try writing it down.

6. Save a folder on your phone or computer for when you are feeling low and want to look over something to lift your mood. I frequently sit and watch videos of my children and the fun times we've had and I also have a folder filled with lovely things that have been said to me by friends, family or on social media and with records of my achievements so I can boost my confidence and remember how far I've come.

7. Take some 'me time' and, by that, I don't mean go for a bath. (I believe I have already covered why a bath is hardly the most relaxing thing a mum can do.) Take the time to do something that you genuinely enjoy. Is it reading? Playing a sport? Writing? Find something that you love, purely for you, not because you make money or because someone needs something from you, and do it.

8. Re-centre yourself with breathing. Ohhh I know it sounds like bullshit, but work with me here! It's a fact that deep, concentrated breathing can make a world of difference. If you have a smart watch, there are plenty of apps, in-built on some models, that will give you a breathing exercise for one minute. If not, you can breathe in through your nose for four counts and breathe out through your mouth for four counts, filling up your chest as you breathe in, and releasing and relaxing your shoulders with each breath out.

9. Accept what you can't change and learn to let it go. If you can't change something, then stop trying. Life isn't always about fixes, sometimes it's about rolling with it. It can be the hardest but the most worthwhile thing you can do.

notes

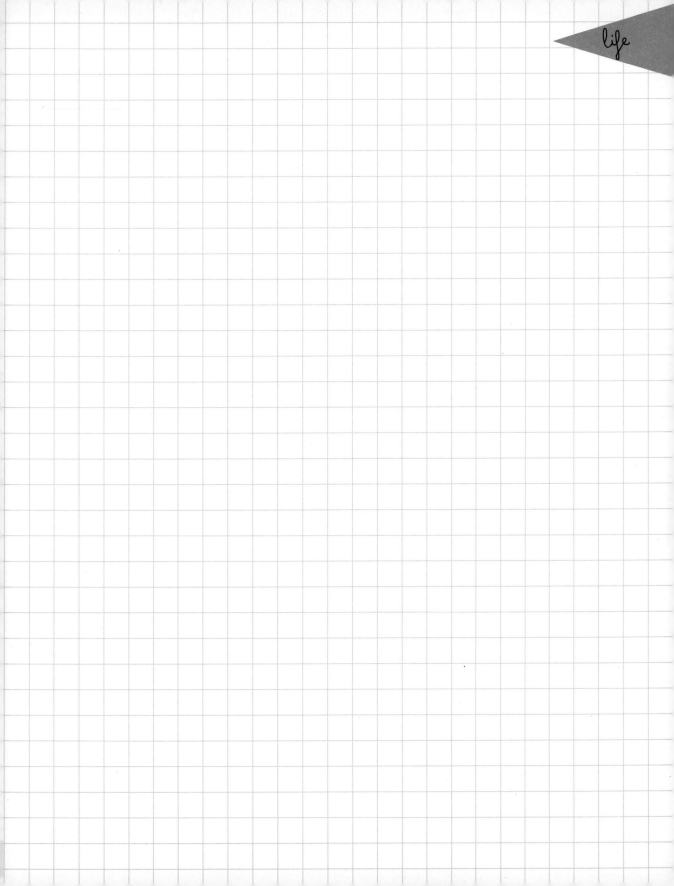

life

The end.

Just kidding, well sort of. This is the end to the book but, unlike a fairy tale, I thought I would finish up with a bit more than 'The End' because, well, life **isn't** a fairy tale.

The problem with fairy tales is that they sell us the dream but never the reality of 'happily ever after'. I mean, what happens when you have to actually live with the Prince, raise kids and deal with the everyday pressures of life? If they did show us the reality of 'happily ever after', I doubt we would love them as much as we do. No one talks about what happened to Cinderella after she got married and discovered Charming's snoring made her want to set Jaq and the rest of the mice on him. **No one shares how she coped with cracked nipples and feet that suddenly didn't fit into the glass slippers because of water retention.**

Being a mum can be really hard at times, especially in our modern age when there are so many other pressures and we're so busy juggling all the balls that we forget to focus on ourselves. If this book gives you anything, I truly hope that it's a bit more time to concentrate on yourself and the faith to believe in your own abilities as a mother and a woman, as well as a bit of a boost knowing you are not alone.

There is no blueprint for this life thing and so we're all winging it. Some days we flourish and other days we try to put the laundry in the dishwasher.

So, there you have it. Now you know what I know about the reality of 'happily ever after...' at least until the kids get to their teen years and then, well, I'll just have to write another book.

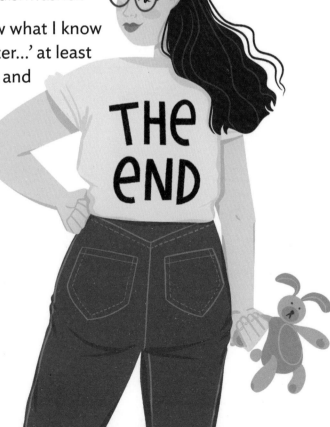

Meal plan

DATE

MONDAY

TUESDAY

WEDNESDAY

THURSDAY

FRIDAY

SATURDAY

SUNDAY

Meal plan

DATE

MONDAY

TUESDAY

WEDNESDAY

THURSDAY

FRIDAY

SATURDAY

SUNDAY

PICTURE CREDITS

Illustrations by Amy Blackwell.

All food photography and styling
by Helen Bratby.

Pages 10, 66, 76, 79 chalks, 84
sponge, 86 grapefruit, 87 shaving
foam, 90 spray bottle, 92 blood,
93 ketchup, 100, 125, 150, 155, 160
and 174, all Shutterstock.

Page 80 Scandiborn. Page 81
clockwise from top left: La
Redoute, Smallable, MADE,
Ikea, H&M Home, Alex and Alexa,
Smallable, John Lewis.

Page 109 © Can Stock Photo/
Mediagram.

All other cutout photography
by Helen Bratby.

All Instagram images by
Harriet and Adam Shearsmith.

S	D	O	U	B	T	R	Y	A	K	B	E	Z	W
C	E	H	X	I	E	R	C	S	G	N	I	G	U
V	N	L	T	P	H	E	S	C	U	O	M	I	S
U	X	O	F	R	U	S	T	R	A	T	E	D	Y
C	J	C	A	S	P	T	E	Q	T	I	O	R	H
R	B	X	I	E	A	F	G	K	C	M	C	D	R
I	N	Y	L	Q	W	B	S	H	Y	E	F	L	T
T	Z	V	I	A	E	A	O	X	V	W	N	V	U
I	C	S	N	M	U	D	A	T	R	U	S	T	Y
C	O	A	G	H	J	M	T	S	A	O	N	E	M
I	P	M	K	M	C	U	D	U	F	G	C	S	T
S	G	B	C	L	I	M	S	M	P	O	E	D	I
M	I	S	S	I	N	G	O	U	T	H	G	C	N
S	U	I	M	P	O	S	S	I	B	L	E	W	F

Acknowledgements

When I first had the idea of writing a book, I almost completely convinced myself that I shouldn't for a variety of reasons and without these people, I can say with certainty that you wouldn't be reading this today.

To my husband, Adam. Forever my sounding board, my first port of call when I'm stressed or struggling to cope with something, all whilst being my biggest cheerleader. We joke that you read me like a book because you always know what I'm feeling, so I've gone ahead and written one. Thank you for always being by my side, even through the tough times. Infinity x infinity. End of.

To my beautiful children, without you, none of this would exist. I wanted to build a career around you so that we could always be together whilst you were little and I could be there for you. Now I have written this for you so that I can give you something tangible to hold. Thank you for inspiring me.

To Craig, Siobhan, Louis and Alex, thank you for being the best management team I could ask for, but also for being my friends. You've always been there to push me, encourage me and never allow me to doubt myself for too long. Craig, thank you for telling me to just write the book and for putting up with me for the last four years of 'I really want to write a book but...' I did it! I wouldn't have done it without you. Siobhan, thank you for always holding my hand and seeing me through the lowest lows and the highest highs.

To my publishers, thank you for believing in me and taking the leap with me. Thank you for supporting me in bringing this book to fruition in exactly the way I wanted to.

To Helen, thank you for seeing my creative vision for the book and elevating it to something elegant and modern, and for the hours of research you put into making the book as beautiful as it is.

To Amy, thank you for such stunning illustrations throughout the book. It is everything I could have hoped for and more, I am so honoured to have you involved.

To Chris, Bec, Maria and Freya, thank you for all your support, your counsel and your belief in me.

To my Toby&Roo community, thank you from the bottom of my heart. Thank you for being there, for supporting me in ways that many of you will never have even realised you do. Motherhood can be isolating and hard, but whenever it has been you've been there in my phone. When I've been through times of self-doubt, marriage troubles, daily life woes – you've been there. Day in, day out for almost a decade. Thank you for giving me the opportunity to realise my dreams and the courage to live them.

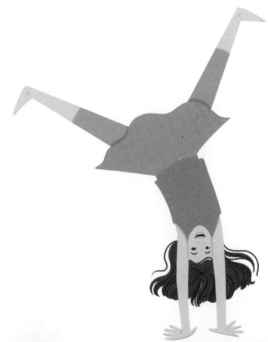